"Well meant protectiveness gradually undermines any autonomy."

Ellen Langer
Mindfulness

Tatiana Fonseca de Freitas

About the Author

JEANNE A. BOSCHERT

Jeanne A. Boschert has been a registered nurse since 1986 and has held a variety of leadership roles within health care. Since 1999, Jeanne has written and developed programs and training materials for a variety of health care providers, including a 40-hour case management training program, a feeding assistant program, and a competency-based curriculum for both nurse assistants and licensed staff in long term care. These materials focus on providing quality of care to the whole person while continuing to enhance the individual's quality of life.

As the Director of Clinical Education for Signature Healthcare in Louisville, Kentucky from 2009 until 2013, Jeanne was responsible for the development of clinical education and professional development programs for facilities throughout seven states. She managed the CEU certification program and worked closely with the education department on content development and training for all clinical staff within the organization.

Currently, she serves as the Director of Operations for the Homecare Division of Signature Healthcare. She is responsible for the daily operations for the state of Tennessee and for the implementation of private duty services into Signature HomeNow divisions in Florida.

In 2010, AHCA selected Jeanne as the author of the fifth edition of *How to be a Nurse Assistant*. The opportunity allowed her to apply her knowledge of clinical education and her experience in health care within a complete program including the textbook, workbook, and instructor's manual. Jeanne is once again honored to partner with AHCA and excited to contribute to the sixth edition of *How to Be a Nurse Assistant*.

Contents

3 INTRODUCTION

4 CHAPTER 1: WHERE YOU WORK

8 CHAPTER 2: STARTING YOUR JOB: WHAT TO EXPECT

13 CHAPTER 3: UNDERSTANDING PEOPLE

17 CHAPTER 4: UNDERSTANDING PEOPLE'S RIGHTS

22 CHAPTER 5: THE NURSE ASSISTANT'S ROLE IN QUALITY OF LIFE

26 CHAPTER 6: THE ROLE OF THE FAMILY

30 CHAPTER 7: COMMUNICATION

34 CHAPTER 8: DOCUMENTATION PRINCIPLES AND PROCEDURES

38 CHAPTER 9: PREVENTION AND CONTROL OF INFECTION

43 CHAPTER 10: PERSONAL INJURY PREVENTION AND PROTECTION

47 CHAPTER 11: THE AGING PROCESS AND DISEASE MANAGEMENT

55 CHAPTER 12: THEMES OF CARE

59 CHAPTER 13: GATHERING INFORMATION

64 CHAPTER 14: THE IMPORTANCE OF CREATING A HOME

68 CHAPTER 15: LEARNING TO POSITION AND MOVE CORRECTLY

73 CHAPTER 16: PERSONAL CARE

78 CHAPTER 17: ASSISTING WITH NUTRITION

82 CHAPTER 18: ASSISTING WITH ELIMINATION

86 CHAPTER 19: MAINTAINING AND IMPROVING SKIN INTEGRITY

91 CHAPTER 20: EMERGENCY CARE

95 CHAPTER 21: PAIN MANAGEMENT, SLEEP, AND COMFORT

100 CHAPTER 22: END OF LIFE

104 CHAPTER 23: OTHER WORK ENVIRONMENTS AND RESIDENT POPULATIONS

114 CHAPTER 24: SPECIALTY SKILLS FOR SUBACUTE ENVIRONMENTS

117 CHAPTER 25: CARE OF THE PERSON HAVING SURGERY

120 CHAPTER 26: SPECIAL SKILLS FOR SPECIAL TIMES

123 CHAPTER 27: RESTORATIVE ACTIVITIES

127 CHAPTER 28: PULLING IT ALL TOGETHER

132 CHAPTER 29: PROMOTING YOUR OWN HEALTH

136 CHAPTER 30: HOW TO BE A SUCCESSFUL EMPLOYEE

140 CHAPTER 31: CUSTOMER SERVICE

143 CHAPTER 32: UNDERSTANDING THE SURVEY PROCESS

147 PRACTICE EXAM

153 SKILLS CHECKLISTS

TO THE STUDENT:

This workbook is designed to be used as a study guide to help you learn the material you are reading in *How To Be a Nurse Assistant*. Be sure to read the chapters in the textbook before trying to complete the exercises in this workbook.

The textbook and the workbook are closely linked, so it is important for you to refer to the textbook as you complete each exercise. Unless your instructor suggests a different approach, work through the chapters in the workbook shortly after reading the matching chapter in the textbook. Answers to the exercises are in the Instructor's Manual.

A variety of exercises have been included in this workbook with the goal of appealing to your individual learning style. Formats include:

Crossword Puzzle
Essay
Fill in the Blank
Labeling
Matching
Multiple Choice
Spell It Out
True/False

Initial activities in each chapter, such as crossword puzzles, fill in the blank, matching, and spell it out, will call upon your ability to find, recall, and be familiar with medical and key terms. True/False, multiple-choice, and essay questions will help you to grasp concepts, relationships, and rules. Labeling activities encourage you to recognize and relate pictures to words. Additional matching activities encourage you to think critically and decide how to handle realistic situations a nurse assistant will face. You will have the opportunity to prioritize activities, choose how to react to a difficult situation, or decide what to say to a resident or family member at an awkward moment.

Take the practice exam, found on pages 147-152, to help you prepare for the written portion of the state competency test. The procedure checklists beginning on page 153 will help guide you through successful completion of all direct care procedures described in the textbook.

Remember that the activities in the workbook are not intended to "test" you but to support what you learn from the textbook and in class. Have fun with these exercises, remember to refer to the textbook when necessary, and ask your instructor for help with any questions you can't answer.

Completing these exercises will better prepare you for completion of the training, successful completion of the state competency exam, and for your role as a nurse assistant.

Chapter 1

WHERE YOU WORK

Using the medical terms below, complete each sentence.

Chronic illness 3
Biologicals 7
Intravenous 8

Occupational therapist 4
Intellectually disabled 10
1 Physical therapist

Recreation therapy 6
Restorative 9
Speech therapist 5

Subacute care 2

1. A(n) _____ works with residents to improve their ability to walk.

2. Residents who do not need to be in the hospital but are not ready to be at home need _____.

3. A condition that does not have a cure, has a gradual onset, and lasts a long time is called a(n) _____.

4. A person who works with residents to improve or maintain their fine motor skills is called a(n) _____.

5. Residents who have difficulty talking may work with a(n) _____.

6. The purpose of _____ is to help residents stay active.

7. A blood product is an example of a(n) _____.

8. Medication or fluids given to a resident through a blood vessel are _____.

9. A plan of care designed to help someone return to health is called _____.

10. A person with impaired mental skills may be called _____.

ACTIVITY 2 – CROSSWORD PUZZLE

Complete the puzzle by using the correct key term from the list, according to the clues below.

Accredit 6
Admission 14
Convalescent 5
Disability 3
Discharge 12
Gerontology 1
Interdisciplinary 8
Linen 15
Optimal 10
Preferences 2
Premiums 7
Rehabilitative 4
Residential 9
Respite 11
Risk management 16
Significant other 13

ACROSS

2. Personal choices or favorites

4. Restoring to former health

6. To recognize a facility that conforms to a standard

8. Involving two or more academic, scientific, or artistic disciplines

10. Most desirable or satisfactory

11. Interval of rest or relief

13. Person who is very close and important to another person (two words)

14. Administrative procedure for entering a facility

16. Process of limiting legal liability (two words)

DOWN

1. A branch of knowledge dealing with aging

3. Lack of a full physical or mental functioning

5. Recovering health and strength gradually after sickness or illness

7. Payments for insurance policies

9. Long term care facility where people live day and night

12. Administrative procedure for leaving a facility

15. Sheets, pillow cases, and mattress covers

ACTIVITY 3 – MULTIPLE CHOICE

Circle the letter beside the best answer.

1. Rehabilitative services specialize in:
   A. Medication administration.
   B. Exercise.
   C. Care planning.
   D. Tube feeding.

2. Subacute facilities provide specialized services for people who need:
   A. High levels of nursing care.
   B. Treatment for HIV or AIDs.
   C. Long term rehab for a head injury.
   D. Supervision so they won't wander.

3. People enter long term care facilities for:
   A. Rehabilitation.
   B. Supportive care.
   C. Many different reasons.
   D. High level nursing services.

4. What is the value of an interdisciplinary team approach to resident care?
   A. People enjoy being members of a team.
   B. One person doesn't have to do all the work.
   C. Information is shared and care is coordinated.
   D. Co-workers have a chance to chat with each other.

5. What does CMS stand for?
   A. Center for Medical Services
   B. Corporation for Medical Strategies
   C. Comprehensive Major Medical Supply
   D. Centers for Medicare and Medicaid Services

ACTIVITY 4 – TRUE/FALSE

In the space provided, write T for true or F for false.

1. __F__ Everyone believes life is worth living as long as they have enough money.

2. __F__ Life ends when a person enters long term care.

3. __T__ The resident's care plan is used daily by the interdisciplinary team.

4. __F__ The social worker is usually responsible for admitting a new resident.

5. __F__ About half of all residents pay for long term care out of their savings.

6. __T__ Medicaid pays for long term care costs for people with limited income.

7. __T__ All long term care facilities provide dietary and pharmacy services.

8. __T__ CMS requires long term care facilities to follow government rules and regulations.

9. __F__ Long term care facilities are surveyed by the state every five years.

10. __T__ All long term care facilities are accredited by JCAHO.

ACTIVITY 5 – IN YOUR OWN WORDS

1. Describe what makes life worth living for you.

Have a religion, being close my family and friends, have time to relax, & do what I like.

2. Imagine what it must be like to live in a long term care facility. Describe how you would feel if you were a resident.

Receiving respect, being treatment with dignity

3. Make a list of things you would like to continue to do if you were a resident in a long term care facility.

Listening music, have privacity, making friends, being independent

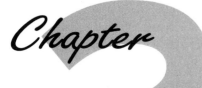

Chapter 2

STARTING YOUR JOB: WHAT TO EXPECT

ACTIVITY 1 – MATCHING

In the space provided, write the letter of the correct definition.

Term	Definition
1. H Ethics	R A. To revive from apparent death
2. D Mindful	S B. Scheduled period of work for a group of people
3. G Contracture	W C. Separate section of a building attached to a central section
4. E Values	M D. Continually being aware _consciente_
5. I Culture	V E. Beliefs people have about what is important to them
6. A Resuscitate	R F. Pattern of activities you set with each resident individually, something repeated
7. B Shift _troca_	C G. A deformity caused by permanent shortening of a muscle or by scar tissue
8. F Routine	E H. Knowledge, awareness, or study of good and bad, right and wrong, and moral duty
9. C Wing _(a sante)_	I. The customary beliefs, social forms, and traits of a racial, social, or religious group

ACTIVITY 2 – TRUE/FALSE

Write T for True or F for False in the blank provided.

1. __T__ A nurse assistant who provides care quickly is mindful.

2. __T__ Our culture influences what foods we like, the clothes we wear, and how we worship.

3. __T__ You gain a resident's trust by being reliable, respectful, caring, and honest.

4. __F__ Nurse assistants are usually too busy to be concerned with residents' likes and dislikes.

5. __F__ Mindful caregiving means making the effort to observe residents closely.

6. __T__ Being on time for work helps show you are a reliable team member.

7. __F__ For most people, stress is usually caused by financial concerns.

8. __T__ The best way to cope with your emotions is to work through them on your own.

9. __T__ An important way to get along with residents and co-workers is to respect their opinions and beliefs.

10. __F__ Factors that influence care include break times and rainy days.

ACTIVITY 3 – MULTIPLE CHOICE

Circle the letter beside the best answer.

1. The term mindful caregiving means to:
   A. Provide care as quickly as possible.
   B. Give care in a thoughtful, efficient way.
   C. Always mind residents and their families.
   D. Spend an hour with each resident each day.

2. You balance the science of nursing with the art of caregiving when you:
   A. Find creative ways to get everything done.
   B. Make sure the resident's pants and shirt match.
   C. Pretend to listen to the resident as you give care.
   D. Talk with a resident as you give them a bed bath.

3. In order to have a good relationship with the charge nurse, you should:
   A. Offer to take her to lunch each week.
   B. Say nice things about her to all other staff.
   C. Be reliable, trustworthy, and communicate openly.
   D. Give her a present on her birthday and all major holidays.

4. A resident who is not assigned to you needs help toileting. You should:
   A. Tell them you are not their nurse assistant and walk away.
   B. Tell the resident to wait while you find their nurse assistant.
   C. Assist them with toileting then tell the other nurse assistant.
   D. Yell down the hall for the nurse assistant caring for that resident.

5. If you're not sure how to do an assignment, you should:
   A. Ask the housekeeper if she can help you.
   B. Talk to the charge nurse about your concerns.
   C. Do the best you can and hope it turns out O.K.
   D. Ask the resident how they think it should be done.

ACTIVITY 4 – MATCHING

Read each example and decide which term it reflects. Write the first letter of that term in the space provided. Refer to examples in the text-book if necessary.

Term

Culture   Ethics   Values

Example

1. __V__ Mrs. DiCaprio has dressed in black every day since her husband died.

2. __E__ Mr. Marlow's family has decided he should not be resuscitated if cardiac arrest happens.

3. __V__ Mrs. Henderson always wants to look perfect before she leaves her room.

4. __V__ Mr. Mooney doesn't want any special measures taken to keep him alive.

5. __C__ Mrs. Logan reads the Bible every morning.

6. __V__ Mrs. Anders was a volunteer for the Humane Society. She enjoys it when pets are brought into the facility.

7. __C__ A member of Mrs. Nguyen's family brings her sushi at least once a week.

8. __V__ You believe in providing the best care you can.

ACTIVITY 5 – YES OR NO

Read each example of caregiving. In the space provided, write YES if it is mindful caregiving, or NO if it is not.

1. __Y__ You listen to Mr. Morricone's preferences about his personal care and do exactly what he wants within safe limits.

2. __N__ Mrs. Baker says she doesn't feel well today and doesn't want to walk. You tell her she needs to walk anyway.

3. __N__ Mrs. Lawler is slow and confused today. You can't waste time, so you rush her along so that you can get to the next resident on your list.

4. __Y__ Mrs. Lim is very quiet today. You ask her if anything is bothering her.

5. __Y__ When you give Mr. Burrell his bath, you notice a red spot on his elbow. You report it to the charge nurse.
cotovelo

6. __N__ Because you are running behind schedule, you pick Mrs. O'Hara's outfit instead of waiting for her to do so.

7. __Y__ As you help Mr. Quinn with his personal care, you ask him the latest news about his grandchildren.

8. __Y__ The daughter of a new resident is visiting today. You stop to talk with her and ask questions about her mother's preferences.

9. __Y__ Even though Mrs. Bradley says nothing is wrong, she seems flushed. You tell the charge nurse.
corado

10. __N__ Mr. Kayser asks you to find a newspaper for him just as your shift is ending. Without looking for one, you tell him they've all been thrown away.

ACTIVITY 6 – MATCHING

Next to each situation, write the letter of the correct response.

Situation	Response
1. _D_ Mrs. Kelly complains that she is in pain. You think people should be able to live with a little pain.	A. Let the nurse assistant know, in a friendly way, that her voice is a little too loud.
2. _B_ Mr. Daly's family has decided he should not have a feeding tube, even though he can no longer swallow. This decision is against your religious beliefs.	B. It would be wrong to impose your beliefs on the resident. Spiritual beliefs and practices are very personal.
3. _F_ A resident never attends Sunday morning services, even though she is Christian. You think she needs spiritual guidance.	C. Don't let the family know you disapprove. Discuss you feelings with the charge nurse.
4. _G_ A resident is asking you personal questions about her new roommate.	D. Put your own values aside. Ask the resident what hurts and tell the charge nurse promptly.
5. _A_ Another nurse assistant on your shift talks so loudly residents have complained to you.	E. In a friendly way, bring up your concerns to the co-worker. Suggest that the two of you discuss work assignments with the charge nurse.
6. _C_ Mrs. Greer believes Halloween is sinful and has criticized staff for making a big deal of it.	F. Remember that she is entitled to her beliefs. Respect her point of view.
7. _E_ A co-worker has been asking for your help so often that you have to rush personal care for your own residents.	G. You explain that you aren't allowed to share personal information about any resident.

ACTIVITY 7 – IN YOUR OWN WORDS

In the space provided, describe why you think it is important to have a good relationship with the charge nurse and your co-workers.

Part A

The charge nurse can assist you to:

1.

2.

3.

4.

Part B

Your co-workers can assist you to:

1.

2.

3.

4.

ACTIVITY 8 – IN YOUR OWN WORDS

What kinds of questions should you ask the charge nurse when you get an assignment?

What can you do to develop a trusting relationship with your charge nurse?

Chapter 3

UNDERSTANDING PEOPLE

ACTIVITY 1 – FILL IN THE BLANK

Using the correct medical or key term listed below, complete each sentence.

Amputation 9
4 Assertive
Generativity 8

Gross motor skills 6
Hierarchy 1
Integrity 7

Psychosocial 10
Recognition 5
Status 3

Theory 2

1. Abraham Maslow believed we all develop needs in a certain order, called _____.

2. When scientists aren't able to explain something, they try to come up with a set of principles or ideas, called a(n) _____.

3. When we have accomplished *realizado* something very important, we want ___*Status*___ by our peers. *elevar*

4. A person who behaves in a confident way is _____.

5. If a middle-aged person feels they have created or accomplished *realizado* something with their life, they have had success in experiencing _____.

6. The ability to run, walk, or catch a ball involves the use of _____ _____ _____.

7. If a resident receives respect and recognition from others, they have _____.

8. A sense of feeling fulfilled, whole, or complete is called ego _____.

9. A resident who has had an arm or leg cut off due to disease or injury has had a(n) _____.

10. Issues that affect our mental and emotional health are called _____ issues.

ACTIVITY 2 – MULTIPLE CHOICE

Circle the letter beside the best answer.

1. Erikson believed the older adult needs to feel:
   A. They are still independent.
   B. They have lived successfully.
   C. They have created a work of art.
   D. They have made the world a good place.

2. Maslow believed that our higher level needs cannot be met:
   A. Unless all lower level needs are met.
   B. Unless we are living with our families.
   C. Until we have more food than we need.
   D. Until we have a lot of money in the bank.

3. You can help a resident meet their need for status by:
   A. Showing them respect.
   B. Changing their bed linens.
   C. Giving the resident a foot rub.
   D. Ensuring they eat a good breakfast.

4. A resident is being visited by their spouse and they want privacy. You should:
   A. Leave the door to the room open.
   B. Respect their desire to be alone together.
   C. Tell them they are not allowed to have sex.
   D. Report this information to the charge nurse.

5. We all have a basic need to:
   A. Remain independent.
   B. Achieve success at sports.
   C. Write the story of our life.
   D. Learn to speak another language.

ACTIVITY 3 – MATCHING

Match each basic need with an example in which that need is involved. Some needs will be used more than once.

Need

A. Physical   1
B. Safety and Security   2
C. Social   3
D. Status   4
E. Self-fulfillment   5

Example

1. A   Responding to a resident who needs help getting to their bathroom.

2. C   A resident shares photos from his many trips abroad with other residents.   Social   C

3. _____   Seeing that a resident gets their dinner tray on time.   A

4. C   A resident enjoying a visit with her great-grandchildren.   C

5. B   Assisting the resident when they use the toilet.   B

6. _____   Wiping up a spill in the hallway of the facility.   B   *derramar*

7. _____   A resident knows that she will not be harmed in any way.   B   *prejudicado*

8. _____   A resident having a book of poetry published.   D

9. _____   Cutting meat for a resident with right-sided weakness.   A

10. _____   Helping a resident with grooming before a party.   C –A   *preparação*

ACTIVITY 4 – LABEL THE DIAGRAM

Using the list of needs in Activity 3, label each level of the pyramid. Remember that lower level needs are at the bottom.

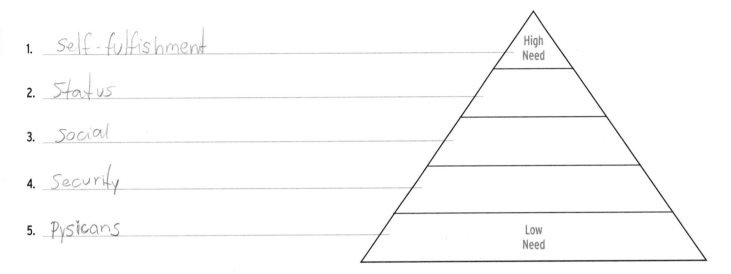

1. _Self-fulfishment_

2. _Status_

3. _Social_

4. _Security_

5. _Pysicans_

High Need

Low Need

ACTIVITY 5 – TRUE/FALSE

Write T for true or F for false in the space beside each statement.

1. _F_ A resident who doesn't attend religious services does not have spiritual needs. ✗

2. _F_ A resident has less independence if you do everything for them. ✗

3. _F_ As a resident becomes more dependent on staff, they may have less self-worth. _valor propio_

4. _F_ A frail or confused resident doesn't have sexual needs. ←

5. _F_ A person's status needs must be met before they can meet their social needs.

6. _F_ If a resident is in pain, their social needs become less important.

7. _T_ Physical needs must be met before status needs become important.

8. _T_ Knowing a resident well is the best way for you to meet their needs.

9. _F_ Once a person has met a higher level need, they never have to worry about meeting a lower level need. ✓

10. _T_ How we feel about ourselves can depend on how others react to us.

1. What activities do you enjoy during your free time? How do these activities meet your needs?

4. List two ways you can assist residents in meeting their physical needs.

2. Think about Maslow's hierarchy of needs. Give an example of an activity typical of how people meet each of the five levels of needs.

5. List two ways you can assist residents in meeting their status needs.

3. How can your understanding of different residents' needs assist you in giving care to residents? Give three specific examples.

6. List two ways you can assist residents in meeting their sexual needs.

Chapter 4

UNDERSTANDING PEOPLE'S RIGHTS

In the space provided, write the letter of the correct definition.

Term	Definition
1. C Advocate	A. weakness *fraqura*
2. B Allegation	B. a person's statement or intended legal action *declaração*
3. H At risk	C. someone who takes the side of another person and speaks for them.
4. L Battery	D. freedom to make your own choices and choose your own actions
5. ___ Confidentiality	E. keeping information private
6. A Frailty *fragilidade*	F. retaliation against or punishment of a person for doing something
7. ___ Hearing	G. failure to do something that should have been done
8. N Incident	H. someone who has a probability of having some type of medical incident
9. G Neglect	I. move to another room in the facility
10. F Reprisal	J. a person's state or situation
11. E Right	K. something one has a just or legal claim to *afirmação*
12. O Securing	L. unlawful <u>beating</u> or use of force *batendo*
13. D Self-determination	M. initial discussion of what happened when charges are made against someone
14. P Sentimental value	N. something happens that is unusual
15. J Status	O. making something safe
16. I Transfer	P. an object of value because of associations and memories it has for the owner

ACTIVITY 2 – FILL IN THE BLANK

Complete each sentence correctly, using the medical terms provided.

Chemical restraint
Circulation
Physical restraint
Sedate

1. Medication that is used to <u>sedate</u>

   a resident or slow their muscle activity is called a

   <u>chemical</u> <u>restraint</u> .

2. Blood flows through our bodies by means of the

   <u>Circulation</u> .

3. A mechanical device used to restrict a resident's movement is

   called a <u>physical</u> <u>restraint</u> .

ACTIVITY 3 - IDENTIFY THE RIGHT

For each example, select the resident right which is involved. Write it in on the line below the example.

2 Right to privacy
4 Rights to information
7 Rights to choose
6 Right to exercise your rights

Protection of residents' personal funds 1
guarda
Grievance rights
3 Transfer and discharge rights
5 Right to be free from restraint and abuse

1. You notice that a resident is giving out small amounts of cash to other residents.

   _____

2. The resident is uneasy *inquieto* and tries to stay covered *cobento* up while taking a bath.

   _____

3. The resident is about to be transferred to another wing of the facility.

   _____

4. A resident's daughter wants to see his medical record and care plan.

   _____

5. A staff member loses their temper and grabs *agarra* a resident's arm.

   _____

6. A resident's family wants to put their complaints in writing.

   _____

7. A resident doesn't like the way a medication makes them feel; they refuse to take it.

   _____

8. A resident wants to maintain contact with friends from her church.

   _____

ACTIVITY 4 – MULTIPLE CHOICE

Circle the letter by the best answer.

1. Residents of nursing facilities have the same rights as:
   A. All children.
   B. All U.S. citizens.
   C. All human beings.
   D. All doctors.

2. Mrs. Ludlow asks to see her financial records and have them explained to her. She is exercising her right to:
   A. Privacy.
   B. Information.
   C. Confidentiality.
   D. Self-determination.

3. A resident must be told that they are to be discharged or transferred:
   A. As soon as staff is told.
   B. One day before the move.
   C. At least 30 days in advance.
   D. At least two hours in advance.

4. Screening of potential nurse assistants may include:
   A. Inspection of their wardrobe.
   B. Checks of family members.
   C. Home safety inspection.
   D. Criminal background checks.

5. Mr. Chang returns to his room and discovers he has a new roommate. Which of his rights has been violated?
   A. Right to information.
   B. Right to exercise one's rights.
   C. Right to notification of change.
   D. Right to privacy and confidentiality.

ACTIVITY 5 – MATCHING

Read the examples of abuse. Place the letter of the correct term for that form of abuse next to the example.

Term

A. Theft
B. Neglect
C. Physical abuse
D. Corporal punishment
E. Involuntary seclusion *segredo / reclusão involuntária*
F. Mental abuse
G. Negligence
H. Verbal abuse
I. Chemical restraint
J. Sexual abuse
K. Physical restraint

Example

1. _C_ A resident is shaken by an angry nurse assistant.

2. _G_ A bed-ridden resident is not turned as often as they should be.

3. _I_ A resident is sedated so they won't wander. *deambular*

4. _F_ Making fun of a resident.

5. _D_ Punishing a resident by slapping them.

6. ___ Locking a resident in a room against their will.

7. _J_ Allowing one resident to touch another in a sexual way.

8. _A_ Stealing a resident's money.

9. _K_ Using a device that forces a resident to remain seated.

10. ___ Making a threatening remark *observação* to a resident.

11. ___ Failing to do what another nurse assistant would do in the same situation.

ACTIVITY 6 – FILL IN THE BLANK

2 Belittles
3 Coercion
Discrimination *5*
1 Grievance queixa
Interference *4*
Ombudsman *7*
Retaliation *6*

Using the word list above, complete each sentence with the correct term.

1. A resident's family wants to file a formal complaint, called a(n) _____ , because of an accident involving their family member.

2. Mrs. Shea has confided to you about an act of _____ she suffered on another shift. The staff member forced her to take a bath when she didn't want to, by threatening to tear up one of Mrs. Shea's family photos.

3. Mr. Logan complained to the nurse about a dietary employee who stole money from his wallet. In an act of _____ . the employee serves his food cold.

4. If you try to prevent a resident or family member from making a complaint, you would be guilty of _____ .

5. Mrs. McDougal has been excited about attending a special holiday event in the activity room. But because she is blind, the staff doesn't take her to the event. The staff is guilty of _____ .

6. When Mrs. Duffy says unkind or hurtful remarks to her roommate, she _____ her.

7. A(n) _____ is required by law to investigate complaints or violations of a resident's rights.

1. Imagine you are a resident in a long term care facility. Which right(s) would you be willing to give up?

2. Describe the difference between a person's needs and a person's rights.

Chapter 5

NURSE ASSISTANT'S ROLE IN QUALITY OF LIFE

ACTIVITY 1 – WORD SCRAMBLE

Unscramble each key term and spell it correctly in the spaces directly below.

Alternative   Dignity   Habitat   Perception   Single-minded

1. Even thought you don't know him very well, you always think of your neighbor as being happy and content. This is your <u>mental image</u> of him.

   ROCPEPTENI   _ perception _ _ _ _ _

2. Instead of going to work the same way as usual, you choose a new route, <u>a different possibility</u>.

   ANETIRVALTE   _ alternative _ _ _ _ _ _

3. Until you saw your boss at the mall with her family last Saturday, you never thought about her having a life outside of work. <u>You only saw her in one way.</u>

   EGLSNI-MEDNID   single _ _ _ _ - minded _ _

4. When you care for Mrs. Fielding based on your knowledge of her needs and preferences and personal history, you <u>convey a feeling of self-worth to her.</u>

   TIGIDYN   dignity _ _ _ _

5. An Eden alternative facility seeks to create an environment where <u>plants and animals are a natural part of the environment.</u>

   THIBTAA   _ habitat _ _ _

ACTIVITY 2 – TRUE/FALSE

In the space provided, write in T for true or F for false.

1. __T__ As a nurse assistant, you influence a resident's feelings of happiness and wellbeing.

2. __F__ New residents will understand if you don't have time to get to know them right away.

3. __T__ Thinking of Mr. Roberts as always being cranky and combative can affect how well you care for him.

4. __T__ Once you've talked to the charge nurse and reviewed the care plan, you know all you need to know about a new resident in your care.

5. __T__ Mrs. Seaver is sad about being in a nursing facility. You can help her by being supportive and allowing her to talk about her feelings.

6. __T__ We are all products of our culture, environment, and life experiences.

7. __T__ The best way to treat a resident is the way they want to be treated.

8. __T__ Staff's perceptions of residents are almost always accurate.

9. __F__ The Eden alternative is a theme park based on stories from the Bible.

10. __T__ Giving a resident a nickname without their permission is a sign of disrespect.

ACTIVITY 3 – MULTIPLE CHOICE

Circle the letter beside the best answer.

1. Your perception of a resident can be affected by:
   A. Their favorite color.
   B. A hot and humid day.
   C. Your own values and culture.
   D. The resident's clothing choices.

2. What is the BEST way to support a resident's quality of life?
   A. Style their hair in a new way.
   B. Knock on their door as you open it.
   C. Treat them with dignity and respect.
   D. Be friendly whenever their family visits.

3. The goal of activities is to:
   A. Keep the activities director employed.
   B. Help residents become actively engaged.
   C. Make decorations for all national holidays.
   D. Give nurse assistants a few minutes of free time.

4. The goal of an Eden alternative nursing facility is to:
   A. Plant flower and vegetable gardens.
   B. Allow residents to care for plants and pets.
   C. Eliminate loneliness, helplessness, and boredom.
   D. Operate daycare centers and after-school programs.

5. What is the most important part of a nurse assistant's job?
   A. Getting everything done.
   B. Meeting all the resident's needs.
   C. Helping the resident get dressed.
   D. Seeing that residents get fed on time.

ACTIVITY 4 – YES OR NO

Beside each example, write YES if the resident's dignity is promoted, or NO if the resident's dignity is not promoted.

1. __Y__ Ask permission before giving care to the resident.

2. __Y__ Call the resident by their preferred name.

3. __N__ Insist that the resident wear an outfit you've chosen.

4. __Y__ Be considerate of the resident's needs, wants, and rights.

5. __N__ Rush the resident through their morning care.

6. __N__ Take the resident to an activity they won't understand.

7. __N__ Treat the resident like a customer.

8. __Y__ Respect the resident's values, culture, and religion.

9. __N__ Leave the door open while the resident gets dressed.

10. __Y__ Take an interest in the resident's stories.

11. __N__ Use baby talk when speaking to the resident.

12. __Y__ Offer the resident choices.

13. __Y__ Ask for permission to enter the resident's room.

14. __Y__ Answer the resident's call light promptly.

15. __N__ Touch the resident's belongings without permission.

ACTIVITY 5 – MATCHING

Match the situation with the appropriate reaction. Write the letter for the response in the space by the situation.

Situation

1. ____ You enter Mr. Galanos' room and, as usual, he has something to complain about.

2. ____ Mrs. Hanak doesn't attend any activities and seems depressed.

3. ____ You have tried before to address Mrs. Lemley's concerns about her meals, even though you don't work in dietary. Today she isn't happy with her lunch.

4. ____ Mrs. Adkins is using a walker today, after having been wheelchair bound for over a week.

5. ____ Your new resident has been very quiet. You learn from his roommate that he is a football fan.

Response

A. As you care for him, start a conversation about football. Encourage him to share his opinions about the sport.

B. Praise the resident for their progress.

C. Remember that the resident has chronic back pain and recently lost his son.

D. Using a pleasant tone of voice, ask the resident what they would like changed about their meal, and work with dietary staff to satisfy their needs.

E. Encourage them to talk. Ask about his/her past, family, hobbies, and talents.

ACTIVITY 6 – QUESTIONS TO CONSIDER

1. Why is dignity important to residents?

2. Describe a situation in which you were not treated with dignity. How did you feel?

3. What do you think happens to residents when they are not treated with dignity?

4. If a resident is unhappy with some aspect of their care, what can they expect from you?

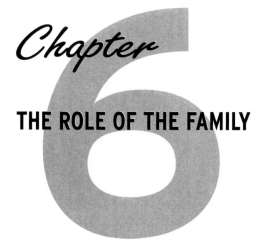

Chapter 6

THE ROLE OF THE FAMILY

ACTIVITY 1 – QUESTION & ANSWER

Read each question. Choose the key term that answers the question and write that term on the line provided.

Family   Feedback   Guilt   Stress

1. When someone has committed an offense or believes they have done something wrong to another person, what emotion might they feel?

   Guilt

2. What is the term for people who are important to a resident, or related to the resident by marriage or ancestry?

   family

3. When someone has a physical or emotional reaction to an event or situation, and that reaction causes them mental tension, what is the reaction called?

   stress

4. When we receive information that is corrective or evaluative, what is that information called?

   feedback

ACTIVITY 2 - MULTIPLE CHOICE

Circle the letter beside the best answer.

1. The family will be happy with the care you provide their relative if they know:
   A. You provide care quickly.
   B. You follow most of the facility's policies.
   C. You provide good care with compassion.
   D. You always greet them with a friendly smile.

2. A family can be an important resource for you because:
   A. They can shop for the resident.
   B. They can bring special foods for the resident.
   C. They know the resident better than anyone else.
   D. They keep the resident occupied when they visit.

3. Each new resident and family goes through an adjustment process that lasts until:
   A. The resident stops complaining.
   B. The family has come to terms with its guilt.
   C. The resident is participating in all activities in the facility.
   D. Everyone is comfortable and a trusting relationship has developed.

4. You will get along with a resident's family if you see them as:
   A. Someone you can socialize with outside of work.
   B. Having total control over the happiness of their loved one.
   C. Someone who should give all the personal care to the resident.
   D. A partner with whom you share common goals and decision making.

5. If a family member criticizes the care their resident has received, you should:
   A. Explain to the family that they are wrong to be concerned.
   B. Tell them to move the resident immediately to another facility.
   C. Listen carefully to their concerns and correct any problems you can.
   D. Assume that they still feel guilty about moving their relative into the facility.

ACTIVITY 3 - TRUE/FALSE

Write T for True or F for False in the blank next to each example.

1. T A new resident in a nursing facility goes through an adjustment process.

2. F The new resident's family always feels a sense of relief.

3. T You should be careful not to judge what a family says or does.

4. T The term significant others means anyone who is important to the resident.

5. F The resident is your only customer, not the family.

6. F Family members are important mostly because they bring in the resident's favorite foods.

7. F Families should not be allowed to help with their family member's care.

8. T Some residents have difficult or stressful relationships with family members.

9. F Families rarely feel sad when their loved one moves into a nursing facility.

10. F Feedback from families is always negative.

ACTIVITY 4 – CASE STUDY

Read the following situations and circle the best response in the following questions.

1. Mrs. Chesnutt, a resident in your care, has emphysema and her health is failing. Her daughter has been critical of her mother's care during her last two visits. She believes staff could be doing more to help her mother improve. What should you say to her?
   A. "I give your mother the best care I can."
   B. "You need to accept the fact that your mother isn't going to get better."
   C. "I can see that you're worried, and I'm sorry you have concerns. Would you like for me to get the charge nurse?"

2. Mr. Lomax is a new resident. He is angry that his family has put him in a nursing facility. When his family members come to visit, he barely speaks to them. What can you say to make the family feel better?
   A. "Mr. Lomax will adjust before you know it."
   B. "This is just a phase. Why don't you put off your next visit until he's had time to adjust?"
   C. "Mr. Lomax is getting the very best care. Is there anything we can do to make your visits more pleasant?"

3. Mrs. White's daughter likes to bring her mother home-cooked foods. But recently the doctor prescribed a low-salt diet, which would mean an end to her meals of collard greens and green beans with bacon. If Mrs. White and her daughter refuse to cooperate, what should you do?
   A. Don't say anything.
   B. Report the situation to the charge nurse.
   C. Remind them about the doctor's orders, but don't insist on their cooperation.

4. Mrs. Cadden's daughter wants to help transfer her mother from the bed to a wheelchair. She insists that the way they did it at home is safer for her mother than the method staff uses. What should you say?
   A. "There is no way I can allow you to do that."
   B. "Let me get the charge nurse so she can review the transfer."
   C. "Go ahead and move her, but the facility isn't responsible if she falls."

5. Mrs. Hearn has just returned to the facility from the hospital. She is weak and must be in a wheelchair because of her brief illness. The doctor's orders are for staff to begin ambulating her three times a day using a walker. Her son is visiting and tells you it is too soon for his mother to be walking. What should you say?
   A. "I'm sorry, Mr. Hearn, but I've got orders to walk your mother. It's my job and I'm going to do it."
   B. "I know you're concerned, but your mother will continue to lose strength if she doesn't start walking."
   C. "I know I'm right about this, Mr. Hearn. I think you should step out of the room."

ACTIVITY 5 – IN YOUR OWN WORDS

1. Think about the most important people in your life. Also think about what it would it mean to them and to you if you had to put them in a long term care facility. How do you think they would feel?

How would you feel?

What would you do to make them feel better?

2. List three things you can do to help family members adjust to the facility and the care their loved one is receiving.

3. How do you respond to families who:

Are uncomfortable visiting

Seem bossy

Are upset

Are arguing with each other

Chapter 7

COMMUNICATION

Complete each sentence with the correct medical or key term.

5 Aphasia
Avoidance *evitaepo*
Clarify *ostlarecer*
Cognitive impairment
14 Collaboration

9 Communication
14 Competition
Compromise
7 Condolences
13 Conflict resolution

10 Context
Curtness
8 Diversion
6 Nickname
15 Nonverbal communication

12 Smirking   *sórrindo*
16 Surname
Tact
Validated

1. An agreement in which both parties agree to give up something is called a(n) _____.

2. Something is _____ when it is proven to be valid, sound, or effective.

3. _____ is the art of saying the appropriate and polite thing at the right time.

4. _____ is a brusque, impolite manner of speaking to someone.

5. When someone has difficulty putting thoughts into words, they have a condition called _____.

6. A person's last name is also known as their _____.

7. Expressions of sorrow or sympathy are known as _____.

8. Anything that distracts a person's attention is called a(n) _____.

9. _____ is the term for sending and receiving messages verbally and nonverbally.

10. Understanding the whole situation, background, or _____ helps to give meaning to someone's words.

11. People are in _____ when they try to beat each other to a goal.

12. The act of working together is called _____.

13. Resolving problems through the use of effective communication is called _____ _____.

14. Escaping from an issue, rather than dealing with it, is called _____.

15. Sending a message without the use of words is done by _____.

16. Family and friends often call each other by special names, called _____.

17. The term for smiling at someone in a way that suggests you feel superior to that person is _____.

18. We _____ something, in order to make sure it is clearly understood.

19. When a person's ability to think, remember, or solve problems has been changed or damaged, they have a(n) _____.

ACTIVITY 2 – DO'S & DON'TS

In the space beside each example, write "Do" if it is an example of good communication and "Don't" if it is a bad example.

1. __Y__ Use a pleasant tone when you speak.

2. __N__ Make eye contact when you speak and when you listen.

3. __N__ Talk with food or gum in your mouth.

4. __Y__ Speak clearly and slowly.

5. __Y__ Use terms that the resident will understand.

6. __Y__ Reduce or eliminate other sounds such as radio or TV.

7. __N__ Roll your eyes.

8. __Y__ Stop what you are doing to listen.

9. __N__ Turn your back on the person you're talking with.

10. __N__ Use medical terms or slang words.

11. __N__ Give residents nicknames.

12. __N__ Cover your mouth with your hand as you speak.

13. __Y__ Validate what the person is saying by nodding or agreeing.

14. __Y__ Clarify what's been said by repeating it in your own words.

15. __Y__ Fold your arms across your chest.

ACTIVITY 3 – MULTIPLE CHOICE

Circle the letter beside the best answer.

1. A confused resident is behaving aggressively toward his roommate. As a nurse assistant, you should:
   A. Run down the hall to get the charge nurse.
   B. In a firm tone of voice, tell the resident to be quiet.
   C. Smile and talk in a friendly voice as you approach the resident.
   D. Approach the resident quickly and pull them into another room.

2. You are involved in a disagreement with a co-worker. In order to resolve the conflict, you should:
   A. Change the subject.
   B. Bluntly say what you feel.
   C. Avoid reacting defensively.
   D. Tell the co-worker they are wrong.

3. A new resident's family is very demanding, and you cannot seem to satisfy them. You should:
   A. Try to ignore their requests.
   B. Refer them to the charge nurse.
   C. Ask the resident to talk with them.
   D. Remember that work will be over soon.

4. If you want to be an effective listener for a resident in your care, you should NOT:
   A. Nod as they talk.
   B. Validate what they are saying.
   C. Maintain eye contact with them.
   D. Encourage them to tell their story quickly.

5. If a resident or family member asks you to talk about yourself, you should:
   A. Share your complete family medical history.
   B. Ask them for advice about a personal problem.
   C. Tell a brief story similar to one the resident told you.
   D. Describe a difficult financial situation you are facing.

ACTIVITY 4 – SITUATION/STATEMENT

Read each situation. In the space provided, write the letter of the appropriate statement.

Situation

1. _____ Mrs. Hooper wants to show you new photos of her great-granddaughter, but you have four more residents to assist with personal care.

2. _____ A nurse assistant has confided to you about a serious personal problem. You don't feel qualified to give her advice.

3. _____ A family member has arrived before her mother has had morning care. She criticizes you about her mother's appearance.

4. _____ Mr. Pierce has kept to himself since he was admitted two weeks ago. You notice that he participated in a current events activity this morning.

5. _____ Mrs. McDonald usually enjoys getting exercise. Today she cringed when you suggested taking a walk to the end of the hallway.

Statement

A. "Are you not feeling well today? It's important for you to tell me if something is wrong."

B. "It's great to see you out of your room. I hope you'll participate in more activities."

C. "She certainly is a beautiful child. I'd like to see all your photos, but I still have residents to care for. What if I come back later when I have more time to spend with you?"

D. "I give each resident all the time and assistance they need to look and feel their best each day. I'm sorry your mother hasn't had her morning care yet, but I have time now to help her bathe and dress."

E. "I know you must be in a lot of pain over your situation. Have you thought about talking to your pastor or a counselor?"

1. What are five ways to promote effective communication?

    _____

    _____

    _____

    _____

    _____

2. What are two specific techniques that can improve communication with residents who have these impairments?

    A. Visual impairment

    _____

    _____

    _____

    B. Hearing loss

    _____

    _____

    _____

    C. Depression or withdrawal

    _____

    _____

    _____

    _____

    D. Speech impairment

    _____

    _____

    _____

    E. Memory loss

    _____

    _____

    _____

3. Describe a situation when someone's non-verbal message didn't match their verbal message.

    _____

    _____

    _____

    _____

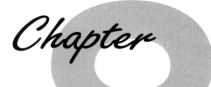

Chapter 8

DOCUMENTATION PRINCIPLES AND PROCEDURES

Complete each sentence with the correct term.

Assessment *avaliaçāo*
Care plan
Documentation

Minimum data set (MDS)
Objective
Quality indicators

Resident Assessment Instrument (RAI)
Resident assessment protocols (RAPS)
Subjective

1. The ___MDS___ contains resident information on the RAI, including levels of physical functioning and bladder and bowel continence.

2. Information is ___subjective___ when it is based on a *pressentimento* hunch you may have about a resident, or it is something the resident tells you they are feeling.

3. A summary of an entire facility's MDS information is called ___quality indicators___, and indicates the quality of care provided at the facility.

4. Any written reports maintained by a facility are called ___documentation___.

5. A written interdisciplinary document, called the ___care plan___, lists the resident's needs and goals, along with the actions and approaches the staff will take to help the resident meet those goals.

6. The ___RAI___ is a tool used by long term care facilities to document key information about residents including their care plans and outcomes. *resultados*

7. An evaluation of a patient or condition is called an ___assessment___.

8. Information that is based on fact, and that everyone will agree with is called ___objective___.

9. The ___RAP___ section of the RAI includes a more detailed assessment of problem areas.

Match the item or type of information with the report or record where that information is contained. Some reports or records may be used more than once.

Type of Information	Report or Record
1. _A_ Needs, goals, and approaches for improving a resident's condition. *aproximar abordagem*	A. Care plan
2. _G_ A description of an accident involving a resident.	B. Flow sheet
3. ___ Admission papers.	C. RAPS
4. _B_ Daily records of a resident's intake and output (I & O).	D. Quality indicators
5. ___ A section of the RAI that has a more detailed assessment of a resident's problems.	E. MDS
6. ___ A summary of statistics about residents and the quality of care they receive at a facility.	F. Medical record
7. ___ Results of a resident's lab tests.	G. Incident report
8. ___ Written guidelines for handling a resident's personal belongings. *pertences*	H. RAI
9. _E_ An assessment of a resident's levels of functioning which is completed by staff in several departments. *de varias*	I. Policies and procedures
10. _H_ Five components including MDS, RAPS, care plan development, care plan implementation, and evaluation & outcome.	
11. _G_ A nurse assistant scraped her arm as she reached for a slipper under a resident's bed.	

ACTIVITY 3 – TRUE/FALSE

In the space provided, write T for true or F for false.

1. N   A resident's medical record belongs to their family. *pertence*

2. Y   The care plan is another name for the medical record. *chart*

3. Y   Physical and occupational therapists may add information to a resident's chart.

4. N   Some facilities use words and symbols on resident's door cards to communicate important information.

5. N   Hunches are based on factual information.

6. N   "This resident is 5'4" tall" is a subjective statement.

7. Y   Good observations should include detailed objective and subjective information.

8. Y   A nurse assistant plays a vital role in the gathering information about a resident's condition. *função*

9. N   The least important assessment tool a facility uses is the Resident Assessment Instrument (RAI).

10. Y   The RAI must be completed for all Medicare/Medicaid residents.

11. Y   "Quality indicators" indicate the quality of care a facility provides all its residents.

12. N   Resident care plans are revised every six months.

13. N   Routine reporting is usually done just before the charge nurse goes to lunch.

14. Y   It is important for you to watch for changes in your residents' health.

15. Y   You should know your facility's policies on documentation before you write in a resident's chart.

ACTIVITY 4 – MULTIPLE CHOICE

Circle the letter by the best answer.

1. The MDS and RAPS are parts of the:
   - A. RAI.
   - B. Care plan.
   - C. Incident report.
   - D. Quality indicators.

2. You should check with the charge nurse before you share medical information about a resident with:
   - A. The dietitian.
   - B. The resident's family.
   - C. The physical therapist.
   - D. The resident's physician.

3. Which of the following items will a typical resident care plan include?
   - A. Graphs or flow sheets of vital signs.
   - B. Needs, goals, and approaches to care.
   - C. Permission forms signed by the resident.
   - D. Progress notes from the occupational therapist.

4. As you talk to a resident about their care, you should always use:
   - A. Hand gestures.
   - B. Correct medical terminology.
   - C. Abbreviations of medical terms.
   - D. Simple terms the resident will understand.

5. What is the proper way to correct a documentation error?
   - A. Erase the entry.
   - B. Use "white out" on the entry.
   - C. Cross through the entry with a single line.
   - D. Cross through the entry with a heavy black marker.

ACTIVITY 5 – SITUATION/RESPONSE

Match each situation with the appropriate response.

Situation	Response
1. _____ Your co-worker has to leave early and asks you to document her residents' conditions.	A. Ask the resident for more details about what happened. Report all this information to the charge nurse so that the right actions can be taken.
2. _____ A resident has made plans to go out to dinner with her family. You're not sure if any forms should be filled out.	B. Make a large "X" over the entire progress note and write "wrong resident" in the margin with your initials.
3. _____ A resident's roommate reports that the resident slipped off the toilet. The resident says "I didn't fall all the way to the floor and I'm okay!" You don't see any bruising or injuries.	C. Repeat your statement using simple terms, "Your doctor wants you to go to physical therapy twice today."
4. _____ You have just written a lengthy progress note in a resident's chart when you realize it's the wrong chart.	D. You are only allowed to document your own actions and observations. Remind your co-worker that it is illegal for you to document for anyone else.
5. _____ You have just told a resident they have orders to go to physical therapy BID. They stare at you and appear confused.	E. You share your thoughts, ideas, and suggestions in a tactful and respectful manner.
6. _____ You are asked to participate in a resident's care planning meeting.	F. Every facility should have a policy and procedure document about residents leaving the facility. Obtain a copy of the policy and follow each step correctly.

Chapter 9

PREVENTION AND CONTROL OF INFECTION

Write the letter of the definition next to the key term it defines.

Term	Definition
1. __H__ Airborne transmission	A. written information sheets describing chemicals used in a facility
2. __D__ Barrier	B. openings in the body where microorganisms can enter
3. __L__ Chicken pox	C. transmission of infection by an intermediate object, such as food, water, medical equipment, or a person's hands, to the portal of entry of a susceptible host
4. __E__ Direct transmission	D. something that impedes or separates a person from an infectious microorganism
5. __A__ MSDS	E. direct transfer of microorganisms from one person to another
6. __C__ Indirect transmission	F. a person, animal, or environment in which an infectious agent lives
7. __I__ Intestines	G. transfer an infectious agent from one person or place to another
8. __K__ Outbreak _surto_	H. route of transmission occurs when the reservoir coughs microorganisms into the air and a susceptible host breathes them into the lungs _pulmão_
9. __B__ Portal of entry	I. part of the digestive tract through which food passes after leaving the stomach; helps digest food and eliminate waste
10. __F__ Reservoir	J. viral inflammation that affects the nerves in the skull and spine
11. __J__ Shingles	K. dramatic, sudden increase in cases of a particular disease or harmful organisms
12. __G__ Transmit	L. contagious disease caused by a virus; one symptom is a low-grade fever

ACTIVITY 2 – SPELL IT OUT

Using the word list below and the definition provided in each example, complete the spelling of the term.

Antibiotics 6
Bacteria 7
Diarrhea
Fungi 15

Gonorrhea
10 Human immunodeficiency virus
14 Immunization
Infection

Sarampo
8 Measles
12 Microorganism
9 Nonpathogenic
Pathogenic

13 Syphilis
Tuberculosis
11 Virus

1. A kind of microorganism like yeast and mold.

F U N G I

2. Microorganisms or substances that can produce disease.

P A TH O G E N I C

3. Infectious, bacterial, communicable disease primarily affecting the lungs, also known as TB.

T U B E R C U L O S E S

4. Contagious bacterial venereal infection that is sexually transmitted.

G O N O R RH E A

5. Condition produced when an infective agent becomes established in or on a suitable host.

I N F E C T I O N

6. Drugs that reduce or kill microorganisms.

_ N _ B _ T _ _ _

7. One-celled microorganisms that may cause infection.

B _ _ T _ R _ _

8. Contagious disease cause by a virus that produces red spots on the skin.

M _ _ S _ _ S

9. Microorganisms that do not cause infection.

N _ _ P _ _ _ _ G _ _ _ C

10. Viral infection transmitted by contact with blood and other body fluids such as semen and vaginal secretions, also known as HIV.

_ _ _ M _ N

I _ M _ _ _ D _ _ _ _ _ _ _ N _ _

V _ R _ _

11. A type of microorganism that survives only in living things.

_ _ _ R _ S

12. Virus, bacteria, or fungus that cannot be seen with the naked eye; also called a germ.

_ _ _ C _ _ _ R G _ _ _ _ M

13. A chronic contagious venereal infection that is sexually transmitted.

_ Y _ _ _ L _ _

14. Administration of a vaccine to make the person immune (not susceptible) to a specific infection.

_ _ _ M _ _ _ Z _ T _ _ _ _

15. Condition indicated by frequent and liquid stools.

_ _ _ I _ R _ _ A

ACTIVITY 3 – FILL IN THE BLANK

Using the terms provided, complete each sentence correctly.

7 Biohazard   9 Emesis   3 Sanitation
4 Condom   2 Invasive   8 Secretions
1 Contaminated   5 Isolation   6 Sterilization

1. If something is impure or unclean, it is _____ .

2. _____ is the term for something that enters the body.

3. _____ is the promotion of hygiene and prevention of disease by maintaining clean conditions.

4. A(n) _____ is a thin, flexible sheath commonly made of latex rubber, worn over the penis to reduce the risk of pregnancy and transmission of sexually transmitted diseases

5. When someone is set apart from others, they are in _____ .

6. _____ causes the complete elimination or destruction of all microbial life.

7. A(n) _____ is anything that is harmful or potentially harmful to humans or the environment.

8. Substances like saliva, mucus, perspiration, tears, etc. are called _____ .

9. A(n) _____ basin is used for vomiting.

ACTIVITY 4 – CHAIN OF INFECTION

In the diagram below, write the six steps/conditions in the chain of infection in the order by which infection occurs.

Microorganism   Portal of exit   Susceptible host
Portal of entry   Reservoir   Transmission

6th _____   1st _____

5th _____   2nd _____

4th _____   3rd _____

ACTIVITY 5 – DIRECT/INDIRECT

Review each action. If transmission of infection could be made directly by the action, write D in the space provided. Write I if the transmission would be indirect.

1. I Coughing
2. I Sneezing
3. I Shaking hands
4. I Changing dressings
5. I Carrying dirty linen
6. I Opening doors
7. D Eating contaminated food
8. D Kissing
9. D Sexual intercourse
10. I Picking up soiled tissues

ACTIVITY 6 – TRUE/FALSE

Write a T for True or an F for False by each statement.

1. T The most important way to prevent the spread of infection is by washing your hands.
2. T It is important to rinse your hands from your fingertips down to your <u>wrists</u> after you've washed them with soap.
   pulsos
3. T Diarrhea is frequent liquid stools.
4. F Protection is not required when assisting a resident with toileting.
5. F Single-use gloves can be reused if they don't look dirty.
6. T A disinfectant should be used to clean up blood or other bodily fluids.
7. F You don't need to wash your hands after a procedure if you were wearing gloves.
8. F If a resident is on isolation precautions, only a nurse can provide their care.
9. T All objects that have been used by a resident or caregiver are considered dirty.
10. T Residents who are on isolation precautions may need emotional support from staff and family.

ACTIVITY 7 – MULTIPLE CHOICE

Circle the best answer to each statement or question.

1. Bacteria is a type of:
   A. Fungi.
   B. Influenza.
   C. Antibiotic.
   D. Microorganism.

2. A microorganism that cannot cause infection is:
   A. Bacteria.
   B. Antibiotic.
   C. Pathogenic.
   D. Nonpathogenic.

3. Mrs. Reynolds had surgery recently and is at risk of getting an infection. In the chain of infection, what is she called?
   A. Reservoir.
   B. Portal of exit.
   C. Portal of entry.
   D. Susceptible host.

4. Direct transmission of a microorganism occurs by:
   A. Handling soiled linens.
   B. Using a contaminated phone.
   C. Kissing or sexual intercourse.
   D. Eating off someone else's plate.

ACTIVITY 8 – SKILLS PRACTICE

Using the Appendix Skills Checklists, practice the following skills:

Handwashing

Chapter 10

PERSONAL INJURY PREVENTION AND PROTECTION

ACTIVITY 1 – MATCHING

In the space provided, write the letter of the correct definition.

Term	Definition
1. _J_ Biceps	A. Hormone involved in breaking down carbohydrates in the body.
2. _F_ Body mechanics	B. Infection of the liver.
3. _E_ Ergonomics	C. Condition of being in direct or indirect contact with an infectious microorganism.
4. _I_ External evacuation	D. Moving residents to another section within the facility for safety.
5. _D_ Internal evacuation	E. Principles of using your body efficiently to do something.
6. _B_ Hepatitis	F. Study of relationships between workers' physical capabilities and their job tasks.
7. _C_ Exposure	G. An agent that inactivates microorganisms on inanimate objects.
8. _H_ Standard precautions	H. Recommendations from CDC for facilities to use in handling blood, body fluids, secretions, excretion (except sweat), nonintact skin, such as cuts and wounds, and mucous membranes of all residents to prevent infection.
9. _G_ Disinfectant	I. Moving residents out of the facility to another site for safety.
10. _A_ Insulin	J. Strong arm muscles used for lifting.

ACTIVITY 2 – SAFE & UNSAFE

Read each example. In the blank provided, write an S if the example is a safe practice or a U if it is an unsafe practice.

1. **U** Wait for housekeeping to clean up a small spill in the hallway.

2. **S** Consider your own strength and body mechanics before you move a resident.

3. **U** Respond to a resident's call light when you have the time.

4. **S** Wear nonskid shoes.   *antiderrapante*

5. **U** Turn the hallway lights off at night.

6. **S** Leave the resident's slippers by their bed in case they get up in the night.

7. **S** Consider the resident's capabilities before you transfer them.

8. **S** *dobrar* Bend your knees and lift using your leg and arm muscles, not your back.

9. **U** *aderir, agarrar* Get a good grip on the resident by holding on to their shirt collar.

10. **S** Remove unnecessary items from the resident's room and bathroom.

11. **U** Set up a new resident's radio using an extension cord.

12. **S** *enxaguar* If a resident gets a chemical on their skin, rinse it off with lots of running water.

13. **U** *encostar* Lean an empty oxygen tank against the wall, outside a resident's room

14. **U** *manipular   perigoso* Handle bottles of hazardous chemicals when you don't know their contents.

ACTIVITY 3 – MULTIPLE CHOICE.

Circle the letter beside the best answer.

1. What is the FIRST step in the five-step approach to preventing injuries when caring for a resident?
   A. Follow the care plan.
   B. Determine the resident's capabilities.
   C. Determine the equipment you will need.
   D. Evaluate the success of the tasks you have performed.

2. *discos giratórios* Pivot discs are used to help a resident:
   A. Exercise.
   B. Use a walker.
   C. Transfer from the bed to chair.
   D. Perform range-of-motion exercises. *(amplitude de movimento)*

3. If you enter a room where there is a fire, what should you do FIRST?
   A. Stop and quickly assess the situation.
   B. Immediately remove all residents from the area.
   C. When everyone is out, close the door to the room.
   D. Yell for help and sound an alarm if one is present.

4. What is the hug position?
   A. A policy having to do with affection between residents.
   B. Holding an object or person close to you as you move them.
   C. Two nurse assistants hug the resident from either side as they lift.
   D. A means of limiting inappropriate behaviors between staff and residents.

5. A resident's bed should be kept in its lowest position when:
   A. You are changing the sheets.
   B. You are giving the resident a bed bath.
   C. The resident is resting in the bed or the bed is empty.
   D. Family is coming to visit and there aren't enough chairs.

6. The goal of standard precautions is to:
   A. Prevent residents and staff from slipping or falling down.
   B. Prevent residents from wandering away from the facility.
   C. Prevent the airborne transmission of the cold and flu viruses.
   D. Prevent the transmission of diseases when handling bodily fluids.

ACTIVITY 4 – SHOULD & SHOULD NOT

Read each example. In the blank provided, write an S if the example is a step you SHOULD take or a SN if it is step you SHOULD NOT take in the event of a fire.

1. SN *tentativa* ~~Attempt~~ to put out a fire that is climbing up a wall.

2. SN Attempt to put out a small fire in a trash can.

3. SN Open the windows in a room where there's a fire.

4. N Use oxygen to put out a fire.

5. S Remove residents from a room where there is a fire and close the door.

6. S Yell for help, and sound an alarm if present. *soar um alarme*

7. ___ Open a door when you see smoke coming from underneath it. *fumaça* *por baixo*

8. S Evacuate residents at immediate risk to the end of the farthest wing from the fire.

9. ___ Throw water on a large fire.

10. S Close the door to a room that's on fire.

ACTIVITY 5 – MATCHING

Match each example of safety documentation to the correct term.

Term

1. C Access to Employee Exposure and Medical Records Standard

2. B Material safety data sheet (MSDS)

3. A Incident report

Example

A. A report on an accident involving staff or residents.

B. A sheet that lists a substance's chemical contents, fire and health hazards, use precautions, clean-up procedures, disposal requirements, needed personal protective equipment, and first aid procedures.

C. An OSHA publication explaining your right to see your medical records, a chemical inventory list, and material safety data sheets.

ACTIVITY 6 – IDEAS TO CONSIDER

1. Make a list of safety rules you were taught as a child, or safety rules you are teaching your children.

2. Of the rules listed above, how many do you practice daily?

3. If you do not practice some of the rules, explain why.

4. Give two examples of injuries that can be prevented by following one of your own safety rules.

Chapter 11

THE AGING PROCESS AND DISEASE MANAGEMENT

Match the letter next to each definition with the correct term for that definition.

1. A Endocrine system

2. D Heimlich maneuver

3. E Pituitary gland

4. B Sebaceous glands

5. C Testes (testicles)

A. body system made up of many glands that secrete hormones

B. glands that are located in the dermis and secrete oil

C. the two oval glands that manufacture sperm cells and the male sex hormone testosterone

D. procedure done to dislodge an object from the throat of a choking resident

E. a gland located in the brain that secretes hormones and regulates other glands

ACTIVITY 2 – FILL IN THE BLANK

Complete each sentence using the correct term.

8 Arteries
3 Capillaries
Cerebral vascular accident

4 Circulatory system
5 Coronary artery disease
9 Congestive heart failure

6 Edema
1 Peripheral vascular disease
2 Veins

1. _____ _____ _____ is a condition that causes a diminished blood flow to the arms and legs.

2. The blood vessels that carry deoxygenated blood from the body back to the heart and lungs are called _____.

3. _____ are tiny blood vessels that connect arteries and veins, where oxygen is exchanged for carbon dioxide inside organs.

4. The body system that includes the heart and blood vessels that carry oxygen and nutrients to the body and remove carbon dioxide is called the _____ _____.

5. _____ _____ _____ is a condition that results in reduced blood flow through the coronary arteries, which nourish the heart.

6. Fluid gain or retention, most commonly observed in the legs and ankles, is called _____.

7. When the blood flow to the brain is interrupted (also called stroke), a(n) _____ _____ _____ occurs.

8. _____ are blood vessels that carry oxygenated blood to all parts of the body.

9. _____ _____ _____ is a condition that occurs when the heart muscle weakens and the heart becomes ineffective in moving blood through the body.

ACTIVITY 3 – FILL IN THE BLANK

Complete each sentence using the correct term.

Digestive system 3
Constipation 1
Enema 4
Fecal impaction 2

1. _____
   is the condition in which bowel movement is delayed and feces are difficult to expel from the rectum.

2. _____ _____ may occur when constipation is not treated; hard feces are impacted in the rectum.

3. The body system that provides the body with a continuous supply of nutrients and fluid and removes waste products is called the

   _____ _____.

4. The procedure known as an _____ introduces fluid into the rectum to stimulate a bowel movement.

ACTIVITY 4 – SPELL IT OUT

Using the terms provided in the box, spell out each word beside the correct description.

Blister 4
Dermatitis 9
Dermis 5
Epidermis 3
Integumentary 6
Malignant 2
Mole 1
Subcutaneous 7
Wart 8

1. A colored spot on the body: M O L E

2. Refers to a tumor or condition that tends to spread abnormal cells:
   __ __ L __ G __ __ __ __

3. The top or first layer of the skin: E__ __ __ __ __ __ __ S

4. An elevated area of epidermis containing watery liquid:
   __ __ __ S__ E__

5. The second layer of the skin: __ __ __ M__ __

6. The body system made up of the skin, nails, and hair:
   __ __ T__ __ __ __ __ __ __ __ __ R __

7. Under the skin: __ __ B__ __ __ __ __ __ __ __ S

8. A horny bump on the skin caused by a virus: __ A __ __

9. Inflammation of the skin: __ __ R __ __ __ __ T__ __

ACTIVITY 5 – FILL IN THE BLANK

Complete each sentence using the correct term.

Arthritis 1
Fracture 2
Muscle atrophy 7
Musculoskeletal system 3
Osteoarthritis
Osteoporosis 5
Rheumatoid arthritis 6

1. Inflammation that causes pain and limits movement in affected joints is called _____ .

2. _____ is another term for a broken bone.

3. The _____ is made up of bones, muscles, tendons, ligaments, and joints.

4. Joint inflammation caused by "wear and tear" of the joint is called _____ .

5. A condition in which bones become weak and brittle due to loss of minerals, especially calcium, is called _____ .

6. _____ is an autoimmune inflammatory joint disease.

7. When muscle wastes away, it is known as _____ .

ACTIVITY 6 – MATCHING

Match the letter next to each definition with the correct term for that definition.

1. _B_ Multiple sclerosis

2. _C_ Nervous system

3. _A_ Parkinson's disease

A. a neurological disease that affects motor skills

B. progressive disabling disease that affects nerve fibers

C. body system made up of the brain, spinal cord, and nerves

ACTIVITY 7 – SPELL IT OUT

Using the terms provided in the box, spell out each word beside the correct description.

Fallopian tubes
Ovaries
Penis
Reproductive
Uterus
Vagina
Vulva

1. A muscular canal in the female involved in sexual intercourse, childbirth, and passage of menstrual flow: _____ G

2. Two tubes that carry egg cells from the ovaries to the uterus: _____ L _____ P _____ B _____

3. Organs in the female's pelvic area that secrete hormones involved in sexual function and becoming pregnant: _____ V _____

4. Body system that provides sexual pleasure and allows for human reproduction: _____ P _____ V _____

5. The external structure of the female sex organs: _____ V _____

6. A muscular reproductive organ where the fetus develops during pregnancy; it sheds its lining during menstruation: _____ E _____

7. Male organ of sexual intercourse and urination: _____ I _____

lung

ACTIVITY 8 – MATCHING

Match the letter next to each definition with the correct term for that definition.

1. C Alveoli

2. F Bronchi

3. D Chronic obstructive pulmonary disease

4. G Cyanosis

5. A Pneumonia

6. B Respiratory system

7. E Acute

A. lung infection

B. body system that takes in oxygen (inhale) and expels carbon dioxide (exhale)

C. air sacs in the lungs

D. chronic inflammatory disease of bronchial passages and lungs; three most common types of disease are bronchitis, emphysema, and asthma

E. health problem that begins rapidly

F. right and left airway structures to the lungs

G. a bluish or purplish discoloration of the skin caused by deficient oxygenation of the blood

ACTIVITY 9 – MULTIPLE CHOICE

Circle the letter beside the best answer.

1. A resident who wakes up with swelling and pain in their arthritic knees has:
   A. A symptom of an acute infection.
   B. A compromised immune system.
   C. An acute condition in a chronic phase.
   D. A chronic condition in an acute phase.

2. What is a silent infection?
   A. An infection that lasts a long time.
   B. An infection with dramatic symptoms.
   C. An infection that does not respond to treatment.
   D. An infection that can only be detected through lab tests.

3. Which body system is responsible for maintaining fluid balance and eliminating liquid wastes?
   A. The urinary system.
   B. The nervous system.
   C. The integumentary system.
   D. The musculoskeletal system.

4. How does the circulatory system change with aging?
   A. Brain cells die.
   B. Muscle strength decreases.
   C. Blood vessels become more rigid and stiff.
   D. Chest wall and lung structures become more rigid.

5. The signs and symptoms of cataracts include:
   A. Hearing loss.
   B. Problems with glare.
   C. Blindness in both eyes.
   D. Heightened color sensitivity.

ACTIVITY 10 – LABELING

Label each of the following pictures, based on the body system it represents.

Circulatory System 7
Digestive System 9
Endocrine System (Female) 5

Endocrine System (Male) 6
Integumentary System 12
Musculoskeletal System 1

Nervous System 4
Reproductive System (Female) 8
Reproductive System (Male) 10

Respiratory System 2
Sensory System 3
Urinary System 11

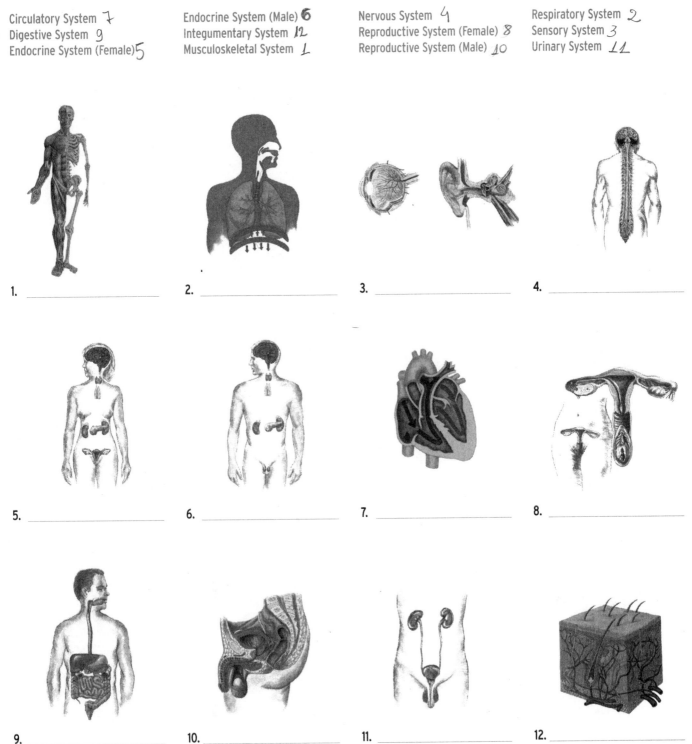

1. _____

2. _____

3. _____

4. _____

5. _____

6. _____

7. _____

8. _____

9. _____

10. _____

11. _____

12. _____

ACTIVITY 11 – SKILLS PRACTICE

Using the Appendix Skills Checklists, practice the following skills:

Collecting a sputum specimen
Application of support hose and stockings
Giving an enema
Applying a disposable incontinence brief
Emptying a catheter drainage bag

Chapter

12

THEMES OF CARE

ACTIVITY 1 – FILL IN THE BLANK

Complete each sentence using the correct term.

Autonomy *3*
Infection control *4*

Maximizing capabilities *2*
Observation *6*

Respect *8*
Safety *7*

5
assunto, tema
1 Theme
Time management *5*

1. A(n) _____ is something repeated over and over.
   Something practiced continually

2. When a resident performs at the level of their own capabilities, it is called _____.

3. A person who is able to make decisions on their own has _____.

4. _____ involves the use of methods to prevent the transmission of infection.

5. The ability to organize activities and perform them efficiently involves the use of _____.

6. _____ is the process of watching and paying attention to details.

7. The theme of _____ relates to being free from harm and secure from threats or danger.

8. _____ is to consider worthy of high regard.
   digno

ACTIVITY 2 – IDENTIFY THE THEME

Under each example, write the letter of the theme it involves. Some examples require more than one answer. Some themes will be used more than once.

Themes of Care

A. Autonomy
B. Communication
C. Infection control
D. Maximizing capabilities
E. Observation
F. Respect
G. Safety
H. Time management

As you help her dress, you talk with Mrs. Jones about her plans for the day.

1. _B_   2. _F_

You use gloves as you handle a sputum specimen.

3. _C_

You plan ahead and talk with the resident in advance of any task.

4. ___   5. ___

You use a guard belt as you assist Mr. Snodgrass.

6. _G_

You encourage Mrs. Fremont to choose what she wears to dinner with her family.

7. _A_

You dispose of dirty items according to facility policy.

8. _G_

Throughout your workday, you make written notes about your residents. Then you use those notes as you do routine reporting.

9. ___   10. ___

Mr. Kent, who is recovering from the flu, asks to choose his clothes and dress himself without any assistance from you. You have noticed that he is stronger, and praise him for doing these things himself.

11. _D_

As you give a.m. care to a resident, you notice that a pipe under the sink is leaking. You clean up the puddle of water, report the problem to the building engineer, and tell staff about it during routine reporting.

12. _G_   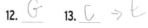 13. _C_ → _E_

As you help to turn Mrs. Scully in bed, you notice a slight redness on the heel of her right foot. You notify the charge nurse immediately.

14. _E_

ACTIVITY 3 – MULTIPLE CHOICE

Circle the letter beside the best answer.

1. **What is a theme of care?**
   A. A special holiday service for residents.
   B. A song that you quietly sing to yourself.
   C. A facility procedure.
   D. A behavior you incorporate into everything you do.

2. **Why are the themes of care important?**
   A. They make it possible to balance your work time and free time.
   B. When you use them, you will always get your work done early.
   C. They help you balance the art of caregiving and science of nursing.
   D. When you use them, you don't waste as many supplies and clean linens.

3. **What is the BEST way to maximize a resident's capabilities?**
   A. Allow the resident to do whatever they like.
   B. Make sure residents enjoy their daily personal care routine.
   C. Work with the resident's capabilities and support them to their fullest.
   D. Always do exactly what the family wants you to do for their loved one.

4. **What is the BEST way to use time management in your work?**
   A. Discourage residents from any changes in their routines.
   B. Try to arrive at work no more than 30 minutes late.
   C. Plan ahead, organize your activities, and perform them efficiently.
   D. Every hour, create a new list of everything you need to do.

5. **As a nurse assistant, your task isn't complete until you have:**
   A. Put fresh flowers in the room.
   B. Checked the next day's forecast. previsão
   C. Checked the resident's environment.
   D. Smoothed any wrinkles from your uniform.

ACTIVITY 4 – SITUATION/RESPONSE

In the space provided, match each situation to the appropriate response and themes of care.

Situation	Response
1. ____ A co-worker is out sick today and you pick up three extra residents to care for. Mrs. Bennet is bedridden and is scheduled for a bath, Mr. Darcy is ambulatory but needs help with bathing, and Mrs. Lucas will need help with buttons and zippers. How can you add these three residents to your schedule without compromising the care your other residents receive?	A. Talk to your co-workers about the resident's abilities (communication, observation). If they think the resident is able to bathe alone, allow them to do so with supervision (autonomy, respect, safety).
2. ____ Mr. Wickham is a new resident who wants to do as much as he can for himself. He is scheduled for a tub bath today, and he insists that he can get himself in and out of the tub alone. You have not worked with this resident, but some of your co-workers have. What should you do?	B. Let the charge nurse know that the resident seems sluggish and weak this morning (observation, communication). Ask the nurse for guidance before you assist the resident with walking (maximizing capabilities, safety).
3. ____ Mrs. Collins is recovering from a stroke, which has caused left-sided weakness. You have helped her walk several times this week, but today you had a difficult time getting her out of bed. How should you proceed?	C. Clean up the spill immediately (safety, infection control). Notify the charge nurse and your co-workers that a resident has had an accident (communication). Check each of your residents for signs for incontinence (observation).
4. ____ Mrs. Phillips has mild dementia. She sometimes tastes or touches the food on other residents' trays. What can you do to deal with this problem?	D. Make a plan before you begin giving care (time management). Check to see that none of your residents has an immediate need, such as assistance with toileting (respect, safety). Let them know you will be back to help them with their baths (communication). Schedule the tub room for any residents you will assist with bathing (time management). Assist the more independent residents with dressing (maximizing capabilities). Ask them if they need additional assistance (respect). Assist other residents with their tub bath. Finally, assist your most dependent residents with personal care, such as a bed bath.
5. ____ You notice a puddle of yellow liquid on the floor. You suspect that it may be urine, but you don't know which resident has had an accident. How do you deal with the situation?	E. Ensure that the resident is not hungry by checking their tray after meals (observation). Offer the resident snacks between meals. Try to watch the resident as trays are being passed out, so that you can prevent any problems (observation). When a problem does occur, be sure to replace the item (infection control).

Chapter

13

GATHERING INFORMATION

Complete each sentence using the correct word(s).

Auscultation 2	Glaucoma 4	Oral 5	Physical examination
Axillary 3	History	Palpation	Pulse
Blood pressure 1	Macular degeneration 7	Percussion 6	Rectal

1. The pressure of blood in the arteries is called _____ _____.

2. A technique of listening through a stethoscope to sounds produced by organs (such as the heart, lungs or bowels) to evaluate a body area is called _____.

3. A(n) _____ temperature is taken in the armpit.

4. _____ is a disease of the eye that can cause gradual loss of vision.

5. A(n) _____ temperature is taken under the tongue.

6. A(n) _____ is an examination technique of touching the resident's body on the surface and more deeply in an organized manner.

7. A condition of the eye that causes loss of central vision is called _____ _____.

8. _____ is a record of a person's medical background, including lifestyle and social information.

9. A(n) _____ _____ is an organized approach to learn about a resident's health status and needs by looking, listening, feeling, and smelling.

10. Tapping on a body area and listening to the sound produced, used to determine if tissue is air-filled, solid, or fluid-filled is called _____.

11. A(n) _____ temperature is taken in the rectum.

12. A measure of the heart rate is called _____.

ACTIVITY 2 – SPELL IT OUT

Using the terms in the box, spell out each word beside the correct description.

Baseline 5
Body Mass Index (BMI) 6
Diabetes 4
Dialysis 3
Policy 7
Protocol 10
Respiration 1
Temperature 2
Trauma 9
Tympanic temperature 8
Vital signs 1

1. Necessary for life: temperature, pulse, respiration and blood pressure: __ I __ __ __ __ __ __ G __ __

2. A degree of heat that naturally occurs in the body: __ __ __ __ E __ __ __ __ E

3. A medical procedure given to some patients with kidney disease: __ __ __ L __ S __ __

4. A common disease involving a problem in the body's production or use of insulin: __ __ __ B __ __ E __

5. Beginning observations used for later comparisons: __ __ S __ __ __ N __

6. A measurement of a person's body fat: __ __ __ __ __ __ S __ __ N __ __

7. A high-level plan for meeting goals, an acceptable procedure: __ __ __ I __ __

8. A measurement of temperature of the eardrum: __ __ __ P __ __ __ __ __ M __ __ __ __ __ __ E

9. A physical injury such as hitting head in a fall: __ __ __ U __ __

10. A facility's official way of doing something, usually put in writing: __ __ O __ __ C __ __ __

ACTIVITY 3 – TRUE/FALSE

Read each statement. Write T in the space provided if the statement is true or F if it is false.

1. **F** To get the most accurate reading of a person's temperature, you should use the axillary method.
   rectal

2. **T** A normal pulse rate for an adult at rest is 60 to 90 beats per minute.

3. **T** You should not use your thumb for taking a pulse.

4. **T** A resident's arm should be elevated above the heart when you take a blood pressure reading.

5. **T** To clearly understand a resident's total physical, psychological, and social needs, a physical examination must be performed

6. **F** A physical examination is always performed by a nurse assistant.
   medical history

7. **T** In history, personal and social information is collected.

8. **T** A nurse assistant should label a specimen immediately after collection.

9. **T** A resident's weight can be interpreted in several ways.

10. **T** Height and weight measurements made at the time of admission are used as baseline data.

ACTIVITY 4 – MULTIPLE CHOICE

Circle the letter beside the best answer.

1. Just before placing a thermometer in a resident's mouth, how should you clean it?
   A. Dip it in a strong disinfectant.
   B. Hold it under hot running water.
   C. Wipe it on your sleeve or a clean gown.
   D. Rinse off the disinfectant under cold running water.

2. Mrs. Buckland's pulse is slow every time you check it. What could cause her to have a slow pulse?
   A. Being angry.
   B. Being relaxed.
   C. Being excited.
   D. Recent exercise.

3. Diastolic pressure is a measure of:
   A. Pressure inside a tank of oxygen.
   B. Pressure inside the facility's water heater.
   C. Pressure in the artery when the heart is at rest.
   D. Pressure in the artery when a person is running.

4. Why does facility staff take a medical history?
   A. To learn about the resident.
   B. To create a care plan.
   C. To get to know the family.
   D. To understand their favorite food.

5. A systematic approach during a physical exam is used to:
   A. Ensure all systems have been assessed.
   B. Make sure the resident has given you all their information.
   C. Let staff feel they have done a good job.
   D. See if the persons family has communicated all necessary details.

ACTIVITY 5 – LABELING

A. Correctly read a mercury sphygmomanometer.

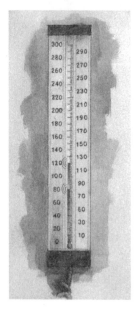

1. What is the systolic blood pressure reading? *blood pressure When the heart is contracting*
2. What is the diastolic blood pressure reading? *blood pressure when the heart is resting*

B. Correctly read the temperature measured by the glass thermometers shown here.

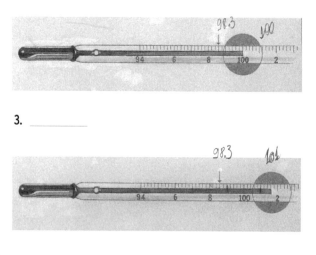

3. _____

4. _____

ACTIVITY 6 – LABELING

Using the list provided, label each photo.

A. Nurse assistant taking a resident's oral temperature.
B. Nurse assistant taking an axillary temperature.
C. Nurse assistant taking a resident's pulse.

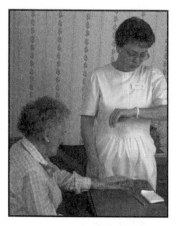

1. *C*

2. *A*

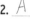

3. *B*

ACTIVITY 7 – SKILLS PRACTICE

Using the Appendix Skills Checklists, practice the following skills:

Taking an Oral Temperature
Taking a Rectal Temperature
Taking an Axillary Temperature
Taking a Radial Pulse
Taking a Respiratory Rate
Taking a Blood Pressure
Measuring height and weight using an Upright Scale

Chapter

14

THE IMPORTANCE OF CREATING A HOME

ACTIVITY 1 – FILL IN THE BLANK

Complete each sentence using the correct word(s).

Adjustment 1   4 Deteriorate   5 Permission   Transfer 3
Dentures 2   8 Occupied   7 Relocation stress syndrome   Unoccupied 6

1. A correction or modification for actual conditions is called _____ .

2. _____ are false teeth.

3. A process that occurs when a resident moves from one area to another is called _____ .

4. _____ means to grow worse.

5. The act of giving formal consent is called _____ .

6. If the bed is empty, it is _____ .

7. _____   _____   _____ is a reaction of an unprepared resident entering a long term care facility.

8. When the resident is in the bed, it is _____ .

ACTIVITY 2 – SPELL IT OUT

Using the terms in the box, spell out each word beside the correct description.

Adjustment 4
Dentures 7
Deteriorate 5
Discharge 3
Occupied 8
Permission 1
Transfer 6
Unoccupied 2

1. The act of giving formal consent:
   __ __ __ M __ __ I __ __ __

2. A bed that is empty: __ __ O __ __ __ P __ __ __

3. Process that occurs when a resident is leaving the facility:
   D __ __ __ __ __ __ __ E

4. A correction or modification for actual conditions:
   __ __ __ __ U __ __ __ N __

5. To grow worse: __ __ T __ __ __ __ __ __ __ E

6. Process that occurs when a resident moves from one place to another: __ __ __ N __ F __ __ __

7. False teeth: __ E __ __ U __ __ __ __

8. The resident is in the bed: __ C __ U __ __ __ __

ACTIVITY 3 – MATCHING

Match the personnel or department with the role they have in admitting a resident.

Personnel/Department

1. _B_ Admission coordinator   B
2. _F_ Dietary department   F
3. _E_ Front office   E
4. _C_ Housekeeping department C
5. _D_ Maintenance department   D
6. _G_ Nurses   G
7. _A_ Social worker   A

Role

A. Help the family with financial issues; sometimes may admit new residents.

B. Primary responsibility for admitting a new resident.

C. Clean and set up the room.

D. Help with move in; may set up phone for new resident.

E. Set up payment schedules.

F. Interview residents to find out their food preferences.

G. Start the assessment process; obtain and confirm all health care provider's orders.

ACTIVITY 4 – MULTIPLE CHOICE

Circle the letter beside the best answer.

1. What is important when making an occupied bed?
   A. Always roll the resident toward you.
   B. Always roll the resident away from you.
   C. Start at the head of the bed and work down.
   D. Transfer the resident into a chair before you begin.

2. When a resident is transferring into the unit, it is important to:
   A. Treat the resident like a new admission.
   B. Wait for them to come to you with any questions.
   C. Bring them candy or flowers on their first day there.
   D. Ask the administrator to give them a tour of the unit.

3. Before leaving the resident, what is the most important thing to do?
   A. Ask the resident if they want water.
   B. Ensure all their pictures are straight.
   C. Remove all soiled linens.
   D. Place the call light button next to the resident.

4. What is the most common reason for discharge from a facility?
   A. Because a resident's condition has changed, a different setting is required.
   B. They don't like their roommate.
   C. They cannot watch their favorite television program.
   D. They can no longer afford care.

ACTIVITY 5 – TRUE/FALSE

Read each statement. Write T in the space provided if the statement is true or F if it is false.

1. __T__ A nurse assistant can make a dramatic difference in a new resident's adjustment to the facility.

2. __T__ A new resident can bring in personal items such as photos, plants, and wall hangings.

3. __F__ After a resident has lived at the facility for a week or so, staff no longer needs to knock on their door before entering.

4. __F__ A draw sheet is used as a temporary screen when a resident's privacy curtain is being washed.

5. __T__ If you find that a call light is not working properly, you should report it immediately.

6. __F__ Discharge from a nursing facility is usually a happy occasion for a resident and their family.

ACTIVITY 6 – CONTENT REVIEW

List five ways a nurse assistant can help a new resident feel comfortable about being in a nursing facility.

1. _____

_____

_____

2. _____

_____

_____

3. _____

_____

_____

4. _____

_____

_____

5. _____

_____

_____

List two fears a resident could have when they are being discharged to a less restrictive setting or home.

6. _____

_____

_____

7. _____

_____

_____

ACTIVITY 7 – SKILLS PRACTICE

Using the Appendix Skills Checklists, practice the following skills:

Making an unoccupied bed
Making an occupied bed

Chapter 15

LEARNING TO POSITION AND MOVE CORRECTLY

ACTIVITY 1 – CROSSWORD PUZZLE

Complete the puzzle using the terms and clues provided below.

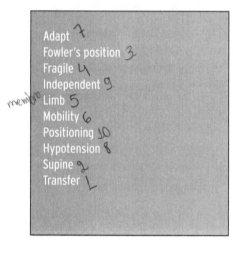

Adapt 7
Fowler's position 3
Fragile 4
Independent 9
membre Limb 5
Mobility 6
Positioning 10
Hypotension 8
Supine 2
Transfer 1

ACROSS

1. move a resident from one surface to another (chair to bed)

3. lying on the back when the head of the bed is raised 30-90 degrees (usually about 45 degrees)

5. arm or leg

7. act of placing or arranging

8. postural _____ means reduced blood flow when sitting or standing, causing dizziness

9. not subject to control by others, not dependent

DOWN

2. lying on the back

4. easily broken or destroyed, delicate

6. capable of moving or being moved

10. change to fit new conditions

front office = payment, apply for medicare and medicate
fowler's position = bed raised 30 to 90°
Supine = on their back with the head of the bed flat.

ACTIVITY 2 – TRUE/FALSE

In the space provided, write T if the statement is true or F if the statement is false.

1. __T__ Someone who has been in bed even for a *short time* may feel stiff or *weak.*
   rigido   fraco

2. __T__ If you don't know a resident well, you should get help before transferring them. *T*

3. __F__ You should never use side rails when moving or positioning a resident. *F*

4. __F__ A resident is supine if they are *sitting up straight.* *T*
   sentado em linha reta

5. __F__ If you position a wheelchair up against a wall, it does not need to be locked. *F*

6. __F__ Postural hypotension causes blood *to pool in the brain.* *F*
   reduced fluxo flow (blood pressure)
   causing dizziness

7. __T__ It is important to have a resident *sit up at the side of* the bed before transferring them to a chair. *T*

8. __F__ A mechanical lift is used to transfer a resident *without the* assistance of a co-worker. *F*

ACTIVITY 3 – MULTIPLE CHOICE

Circle the letter beside the best answer.

1. Why is it important to be careful when transferring a resident who has osteoporosis from a bed to a chair? *propenso*
   A. A resident with osteoporosis is *prone* to weakness.
   B. Residents who have osteoporosis get dizzy very quickly.
   C. Residents with osteoporosis are at risk for breaking bones. ✓
   D. Sometimes blood can pool in their extremities and cause confusion.

2. You are walking Mrs. Reynolds down the hall when she becomes faint and begins to fall. What is the BEST way to prevent her from injuring herself?
   A. Pin her against the wall until a co-worker arrives.
   B. Put both arms around her and drag her to a nearby chair.
   C. Holding on to her guard belt, help her sit down on the floor. ✓
   D. Grab hold of her hair to prevent her head from hitting the floor.

3. You are assisting a co-worker as they move a resident *up in a chair.* Where will your hands be positioned?
   A. One hand on the guard belt, one under their *buttocks.* *nadegas*
   B. One hand under the resident's knee, the other under their arm.
   C. One hand on the guard belt, the other hand under the resident's knee. ✓
   D. One hand under the resident's arm, the other hand around the resident's ankle.

4. Mrs. Desmond has a hip fracture. You have reminded her that she shouldn't cross her legs, but she forgets. How can you prevent her from re-injuring her hip?
   A. Transfer her back to the bed.
   B. Put a pillow between her legs. ✓
   C. Suggest she stand instead of sit.
   D. Call her doctor to report the problem.

5. When you position a resident on their back, their legs should normally be positioned:
   A. With a pillow between them.
   B. As close together as possible.
   C. With both legs straight and slightly apart. ✓
   D. With one leg straight and one leg slightly *bent.* *curvade*

ACTIVITY 4 – SITUATION/RESPONSE

Read each situation. In the space provided, write the letter of the appropriate response to that situation.

Situation	Response
1. ____ Mrs. Saunders has left sided weakness. You have to transfer her out of a wheelchair onto the toilet.	A. Place a gait belt around her waist. Standing on either side of the resident, have a co-worker assist you by pulling up on the belt with one hand and lifting the resident's knees with the other hand.
2. ____ You notice that Mrs. Walters has slumped down in her chair. She is unable to pull herself back up to a comfortable position.	B. Place her in a side-lying position. Stand on the side to which you will turn her. With a hand on her shoulder and the other on her hip, help her turn toward you. Position her head, neck arms, and legs comfortably.
3. ____ Mr. Hudson has been in bed with the flu for several days. He wants to get up and walk to the bathroom.	C. Place a stool or pillow under her feet so that her knees and hips are at the same height.
4. ____ Mrs. Adamson has been lying on her back for almost two hours. You need to reposition her.	D. Position the wheelchair so that her strong side is closest to the toilet. Lock the wheels, raise the footrests, and assist her with a stand pivot transfer.
5. ____ You have transferred Mrs. Adjani from the bed to a chair. She says she is comfortable, but you notice that her feet don't touch the floor.	E. To prevent dizziness, have him roll onto his side and then sit at the edge of the bed with his legs dangling for a few minutes.

ACTIVITY 5 – CONTENT REVIEW

In the column to the left, list five effects that could occur if a resident is confined to the bed. In the right column, list the body system that is involved in the effect.

Effect	Body System
1. _____	_____
2. _____	_____
3 _____	_____
4. _____	_____
5. _____	_____

ACTIVITY 6- IN YOUR OWN WORDS

1. Have you had to sit or lie absolutely still for a long time? How did it feel?

2. Would you feel embarrassed if caretakers had to use a mechanical life to get you out of bed?

3. Have you ever fallen on the ice or while playing a game? Did it hurt? Did it make you more cautious?

4. When would it be proper to leave a resident who has fallen alone?

ACTIVITY 7 – SKILLS PRACTICE

Using the Appendix Skills Checklists, practice the following skills:

Moving Up in Bed When a Resident Can Help
Moving Up in Bed When a Resident Is Unable To Help
Moving to the Side of the Bed When a Resident Can Help
Moving to the Side of the Bed When a Resident Is Unable To Help
Moving a Resident to the Side of the Bed Using a Draw Sheet
Turning a Resident from Supine to Side-Lying for Personal Care
Moving the Resident from Supine Position to Sitting
Moving the Resident from Sitting to Supine Position
The Stand Pivot Transfer
Assisted Transfer with an Assistive Device (One Person)
Transferring a Resident from a Chair to a Bed, Commode, or Toilet
Moving a Resident with a Mechanical Lift
Moving a Resident Up in a Chair
Returning a Resident to Bed Using a Mechanical Lift
Positioning a Resident on Their Back
Positioning a Resident on Their Side (Side-Lying Position)

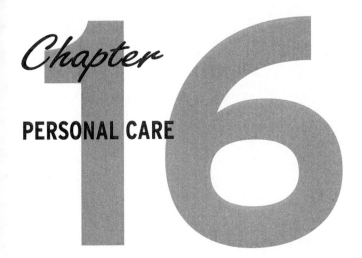

Chapter 16
PERSONAL CARE

ACTIVITY 1 – MATCHING

Review both lists. In the space provided by each term, write the letter of the correct definition.

1. _C_ Anus C   A. an organism of microscopic size

2. _E_ Aspirate E   B. the canal in males and females that carries urine from the bladder; in males it also serves as the duct for sperm

3. _H_ Comatose H   C. the posterior opening of the large intestine

4. _F_ Foreskin F   D. physician specializing in the care and treatment of the feet

5. _J_ Labia J   E. to breathe in or draw in by suction

6. _A_ Microorganism A F. a fold of skin that covers the tip of the penis in an uncircumcised male

7. _I_ Perineal I   G. the external pouch in males that contains the testes

8. _D_ Podiatrist D   H. someone in a coma

9. _G_ Scrotum G   I. area of body between the anus and the posterior part of the external genitals

10. _B_ Urethra B   J. the outer and inner fatty folds bounding the vulva

Using the words provided, complete each sentence correctly.

Antiseptic 4
Corn 11
7 Drape *poner*
2 Lather *espuma*
Objective 1
Observation 15
Penis 16
Personal 14
Perspiration 6
3 Pubic
Stimulate 10
Subjective 9
Therapeutic 12
5 Tolerate
Uncircumcised 8
Vagina 13

1. When something can be observed externally, it is _____.

2. When shaving cream or soap is mixed with water it turns into a foam or froth called _____.

3. The genitals are referred to as the _____ area.

4. A(n) _____ is a substance that reduces the growth or action of microorganisms.

5. If you put up with something or endure it, you _____ it.
   levantar   *soportar*

6. _____ is a saline fluid secreted by sweat glands.

7. When you cover something up, you _____ it.

8. A penis that has foreskin remaining at the tip is _____.

9. Something is _____ if the person feels it internally. It is the opposite of objective.

10. The word _____ means to arouse a function.
    despertar

11. A(n) _____ is a local hardening and thickening of epidermis (as on a toe).

12. The word _____ refers to a treatment.

13. The _____ is a canal in a female from the uterus to the external orifice of the genitals.

14. If something is private, or refers to a person's body, it is _____.

15. _____ is the act of recognizing and noting a fact.

16. The _____ is the male organ of urination and copulation.

ACTIVITY 3 – TRUE/FALSE

Read each statement. In the space provided, write T if the statement is true, or F if the statement is false.

1. __T__ Observing is a major part of your role as a nurse assistant.

2. __T__ It is important for a nurse assistant to report changes to the charge nurse.

3. __F__ Some changes in a resident's status are not important.

4. __F__ A comatose resident should receive oral care no more than four times per day. 2|2 hours

5. _____ Flossing is a healthy habit for all residents.

6. __T__ Before trimming a resident's facial hair, you should check with the charge nurse.

7. __T__ Grooming should always reflect the resident's preferences.

8. __T__ It is OK to trim a resident's toenails if they ask you to do so.

ACTIVITY 4 – MULTIPLE CHOICE

Circle the letter beside the best answer.

1. As you provide personal care, you should:
   A. Change your uniform.
   B. Always wear a gown, gloves, and mask.
   C. Protect the resident's dignity and privacy.
   D. Ask the resident's roommate to stay in the room.

2. Why is it important to wear gloves when you provide mouth care?
   A. In case the resident's gums bleed.
   B. The resident may have bad breath.
   C. So you won't have to wash your hands.
   D. In case you get toothpaste on your hands.

3. When is the bath water changed during a bed bath?
   A. Before washing the perineum.
   B. After washing the face and neck.
   C. After washing the feet and hands.
   D. Any time the water gets cold, soapy, or dirty.

4. What is the correct way to wash the female perineal area?
   A. Wash the anus first, then the labia.
   B. Wash the pubic area first, then the anus.
   C. Wash the entire area in a circular motion.
   D. Wash back and forth over the entire area twice.

5. When you are helping to dress a resident with a paralyzed arm you should:
   A. Put the shirt on the weak arm last.
   B. Put the shirt on the weak arm first.
   C. Put the shirt on the arm closest to you.
   D. Put the shirt on the arm farthest from you.

ACTIVITY 5 – SUBJECTIVE/OBJECTIVE

Read each description. Write S if the description is subjective, or O if it is objective.

1. _O_ While providing foot care, you notice one of Mrs. Russo's toenails is embedded in the skin. O

2. _S_ Mrs. Kramer says her gums hurt when she brushes her teeth. S

3. _S_ A resident seems anxious and upset. S

4. _O_ Mr. Reynolds has a scrape on his forearm. O

5. _O_ An oral temperature of 102.6 F. O

6. _S_ Mr. Dawson said, "I don't want to drink my milk." S

7. _S_ A resident tells you they are in pain. S

8. _O_ Mrs. Curtis is holding her head between her hands, rocking back and forth, and crying.

ACTIVITY 6 – SITUATION/RESPONSE

In the space provided by each situation, write the letter of the correct response.

Situation

1. ____ Mrs. Bertram, a blind resident in your care, is going out to lunch with her daughter. She wants to look her best for the outing.

2. ____ You find a red spot on a resident's hip. It doesn't go away.

3. ____ Mrs. Crawford has limited mobility in her left shoulder and needs help getting ready for bed.

4. ____ Mr. Price has a chronic problem with dizziness.

5. ____ Mrs. Rushworth insists on wearing a yellow and orange floral blouse with red and black plaid pants.

Response

A. Help the resident by unzipping their dress. As you put a gown on the resident, put the sleeve on their left arm first.

B. Suggest the resident sit at the side of the bed as you help them dress. Help the resident to put on and take off their shoes and socks.

C. Help the resident choose color-coordinated clothes. Get the clothes out of the closet and help the resident put them on.

D. Allow the resident to choose what they want to wear.

E. Let the charge nurse know about the change in the resident's condition immediately.

ACTIVITY 7 – SKILLS PRACTICE

Using the Appendix Skills Checklists, practice the following skills:

Complete Bed Bath
Tub Bath
Shower
Whirlpool Bath
Shampooing and Conditioning
Brushing and Flossing
Caring for Dentures
Mouth Care for Comatose Residents
Shaving a Male Resident's Face
Shaving a Female Resident's Underarms
Shaving a Female Resident's Legs
Trimming Facial Hair
Hair Care
Care of Fingernails
Care of Toenails
Dressing a Dependent Resident
Undressing a Dependent Resident

Chapter 17

ASSISTING WITH NUTRITION

Complete each sentence by adding the correct term.

Dehydration 1   Hydration 4   Supplements 8
Dysphagia 6   Nutrition 3   Turgor 2
Esophagus 7   Sodium 5

1. _____ can occur if a resident does not have adequate fluid intake.

2. Tight skin that does not "tent" has _____, which is a sign of good hydration.

3. The act of nourishing or being nourished is called _____.

4. Maintaining an adequate fluid level in the body is _____.

5. _____ is also called salt.

6 Someone who has difficulty chewing or swallowing food has a condition known as _____.

7. The _____ is a muscular tube that leads from the mouth to the stomach.

8. Residents who need additional nutrition may receive it in concentrated amounts through _____.

ACTIVITY 2 – TRUE/FALSE

In the space provided, write T if the statement is true, or F if the statement is false.

1. _____ The food service department provides support with finances.

2. _____ A resident's nutritional status can be enhanced with a combination of correct diet and proper assistance from the nurse assistant.

3. _____ All residents are given a therapeutic diet.

4. _____ A calorie-restricted diet is usually ordered for diabetics.

5. _____ A resident who has difficulty swallowing has aphasia.

6. _____ The food service department uses a feeding tube to mix foods.

7. _____ Intake is the measurement of food and fluids a resident takes in.

8. _____ A nurse assistant measures a resident's weight just to have something to talk about with family members.

9. _____ It is critical to monitor a resident's fluid intake and output.

10. _____ You should notify the charge nurse immediately if a resident's weight drops 1 pound in two months.

ACTIVITY 3 – MULTIPLE CHOICE

Circle the letter by the best answer.

1. Why is it important to "liberalize" therapeutic diets?
   A. So that they will be more nutritious.
   B. Therapeutic diets contain too much sugar.
   C. Therapeutic diets are generally too low in calories.
   D. A person may not eat as much if their diet is too restricted.

2. Renal diets often restrict:
   A. Fats.
   B. Fiber.
   C. Sugar.
   D. Protein.

3. As you distribute meals to residents, you should check to see if:
   A. Each tray has a bud vase and flower.
   B. Each meal includes a serving of red meat.
   C. Each tray has the right diet for the resident.
   D. Each meal has only fat-free, sugar-free desserts.

4. What happens when a person aspirates their food?
   A. They feel like taking a nap.
   B. They throw up their dinner.
   C. They feel the need to belch.
   D. They may develop pneumonia.

5. Which of the following signs is an indication of dehydration?
   A. Sunken eyes.
   B. Good skin turgor.
   C. Alzheimer's disease.
   D. Frequent trips to the bathroom.

6. In order to stay hydrated, a resident must:
   A. Avoid sweet foods.
   B. Keep out of the sun.
   C. Drink plenty of fluids.
   D. Bathe or shower each day.

ACTIVITY 4 – CONVERT THE AMOUNTS

Using these formulas, convert the following serving amounts to cc.

1 ounce (oz) = 30 cc
1 cup = 240 cc

1. A 4 oz serving of orange juice = _____ cc.

2. A 6 oz serving of coffee = _____ cc.

3. A 1/2 cup of Jell-O = _____ cc.

4. A tumbler containing 1 1/2 cups of iced tea = _____ cc.

5. A 3 oz serving of ice cream = _____ cc.

6. An 8 oz bowl of soup = _____ cc.

ACTIVITY 5 – SITUATION/RESPONSE

Match the situation with the appropriate response by a nurse assistant. Some responses will be used more than once.

Situation	Response
1. _____ A resident tells you they cannot cut their meat.	A. Assist the resident.
2. _____ You check a resident's water pitcher and find that it is full.	B. Report this to the charge nurse.
3. _____ A resident ate only 25% of their meal.	C. Obtain the missing item.
4. _____ You pass trays out to residents.	D. Offer the resident water.
5. _____ A resident tells you they are thirsty.	E. Check the tray card and the resident's ID band.
6. _____ A resident cannot open their milk carton.	
7. _____ A tray arrives without utensils.	
8. _____ You are serving a new resident.	
9. _____ A resident says they have the wrong tray.	
10. _____ A resident refuses to eat anything you offer.	

ACTIVITY 6 – LABELING

Identify the percentage of food eaten. Write the letter of the correct percentage by the correct photo.

A. 75% B. 90% C. 25% D. 50%

1. _____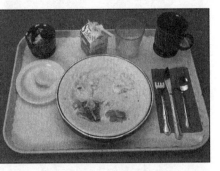

2. _____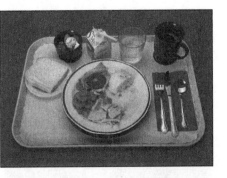

3. _____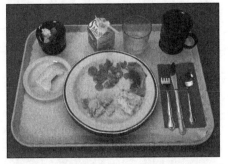

4. _____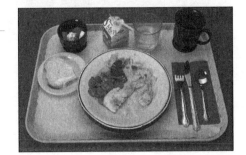

ACTIVITY 7 – CONTENT REVIEW

Write the answers in the space provided. Refer to the textbook if necessary.

Why would residents be placed on the following diets?

1. Calorie-restricted diet:

   _____

   _____

2. Sodium-restricted diet:

   _____

   _____

3. Fat/cholesterol-restricted diet:

   _____

   _____

4. Protein-restricted diet:

   _____

   _____

5. Why would a resident need supplements?

   _____

   _____

6. What is your role as a nurse assistant in assisting residents with meals?

   _____

   _____

Chapter 18

ASSISTING WITH ELIMINATION

Using the list of terms and the clues provided below, complete the puzzle.

Bladder	Gastrointestinal	Occult	Stoma	Urine
Bowel	Guiacing	Ostomy	Stool	Void
Elimination	Incontinence	Parasite	Urinate	

ACROSS

5. related to the stomach and intestines
7. refers to the large and small intestines
8. an organism that lives in or on another organism
10. the process of ridding the body of urine and stool
11. a surgical opening from the intestine to outside the body
12. waste liquid secreted by the kidney
13. a surgically created opening

DOWN

1. procedure for checking for blood in the stool
2. inability to hold urine or stool is called
3. to eliminate liquid waste from the body
4. sac inside the body that holds urine
6. human waste, or feces, from the bowel
9. to pass urine
11. refers to blood that is present in stool but cannot be seen

ACTIVITY 2 – FILL IN THE BLANK

Complete each sentence with the correct word.

Analyze 3   Commode 1   Concentrated 2   Frequency 4

1. A portable toilet, also called a(n) _____ ,
    is a box-like structure with a chamber pot under an open seat.

2. Urine is _____ if it is less diluted, or
    more intense in color.

3. Lab tests are done to _____ the chemical
    parts of urine, stool, or other specimens.

4. _____ refers to how often something
    happens, or a habitual pattern.

ACTIVITY 3 – MULTIPLE CHOICE

Circle the letter beside the best answer.

1. **When should you question a new resident about their elimination patterns?**
    A. While family members are present.
    B. Within minutes after they are admitted.
    C. As you introduce them to other residents.
    D. At a convenient time and in a private place.

2. **Solid waste discharged from the bowel is called:**
    A. Feces.
    B. Urine.
    C. Stoma.
    D. Guiacing.

3. **All specimens are considered to be:**
    A. Dirty.
    B. Bloody.
    C. Watery.
    D. Cloudy.

4. **When is a clean-catch urine specimen collected?**
    A. After a 24-hour fasting period.
    B. After the urethral opening is cleansed.
    C. After the resident has emptied their bladder.
    D. After the resident has had a bowel movement.

5. **An ostomy that routes the colon to an opening on the surface of the abdomen is called:**
    A. A stoma.
    B. A colostomy.
    C. An ileostomy.
    D. A ureterostomy.

ACTIVITY 4 – CONTENT REVIEW

List three ways you can determine a resident's elimination pattern.

1. _____

2. _____

3. _____

Describe four ways you can help ensure that a resident's elimination pattern stays normal.

4. _____

5. _____

6. _____

7. _____

List four ways to help maintain a resident's dignity when assisting them with elimination.

8. _____

9. _____

10. _____

11. _____

ACTIVITY 5 – YES OR NO

For each situation, write Y for yes if it should be reported to the charge nurse, or N for no if you would not report it.

1. __Y__ The resident's urine had a foul odor.

2. __Y__ The resident had a painful, hard, black stool today.

3. __Y__ The resident complained of painful urination.

4. __Y__ The resident's stool had red blood in it.

5. __N__ The resident urinated two times during your shift.

6. __Y__ The resident was incontinent for the first time.

7. __N__ The resident drank two cups of coffee during your shift.

8. __Y__ The resident's abdomen is swollen and they have not had a bowel movement in two days.

9. __N__ The resident's urine was clear.

10. ___falta___ The resident had a watery, foul-smelling stool today.

ACTIVITY 6 – DIGNITY CHECKLIST

Read each statement and indicate if the nurse assistant protected the resident's dignity. In the space provided, write D if the resident's dignity is protected or N if it is not protected.

1. _D_ You respond to a resident's call light immediately.

2. _D_ You close the door before helping the resident use a bedpan.

3. _N_ You tease the resident about wetting herself.

4. _N_ You discuss a resident's bowel problems in front of their roommate's family.

5. _N_ You left the resident sitting on the toilet for 30 minutes.

6. _D_ You talk in private with a resident about their elimination pattern.

7. _N_ You leave a stool sample on the desk, with the resident's name clearly marked on the label.

ACTIVITY 7 – SKILLS PRACTICE

Using the Appendix Skills Checklists, practice the following skills:

Helping a Resident Use a Bedpan
Helping a Male Resident Use a Urinal
Helping a Resident Use a Portable Commode
Collecting a Urinalysis Specimen
Collecting a Clean-Catch Urinalysis Specimen
Collecting a 24-Hour Urine Specimen
Testing Urine for Ketones
Testing a Stool Specimen for Occult Bleeding

ACTIVITY 8 – LABELING

Match each photo with the name of the item. In the space provided, write the letter found next to the photo.

A. Urinal   B. Bedside commode   C. Fracture pan   D. Bedpan

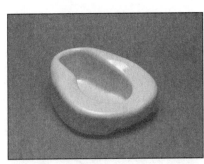

1. _C_

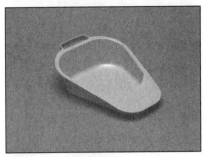

2. _D_

3. _B_

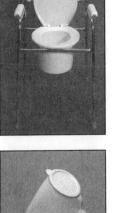

4. _A_

Chapter 19

MAINTAINING AND IMPROVING SKIN INTEGRITY

ACTIVITY 1 – FILL IN THE BLANK

Complete each sentence by adding the correct term.

Contusion 3   Incision 1
Decubitus ulcer 2   Laceration 5
Dermatitis 6   Puncture 4

1. A(n) _____ is a type of wound with straight edges, made by a sharp instrument or object.

2. An opening or wound that appears in pressure areas of skin overlying a bony area in an immobile person is a(n) _____
    _____.

3. A(n) _____ is a type of wound made by blunt force, causing bruising and swelling, but usually the skin is not broken.

4. A type of wound down into the skin, made by something pointed is called a(n) _____.

5. A(n) _____ is a type of wound made by an object causing an irregular, jagged wound.

6. An inflammation of the skin, which may look like redness or a rash and causes itching is called _____.

Write T if the statement is true or F if it is false.

1. T   Even if a person is born with healthy skin, they are at risk for pressure ulcers when they are elderly. ?

2. F   Only a nurse or doctor can identify redness on the skin.

3. F   An overweight person can't develop pressure ulcers.

4. T   ROM exercises can improve circulation.

5. T   As a nurse assistant, you are in the best position to observe the resident's skin from head to toe.

6. T   Daily inspection of the skin is an excellent way to prevent pressure ulcers.

7. F   Stage IV pressure ulcers should be treated only with daily bathing.

8. T   A resident is at high risk for skin breakdown if they cannot go to the toilet by themselves.

9. F   Stage I pressure ulcers have a foul smell or discharge.

10. F   Active people are at greater risk for skin breakdown.

11. T   Cornstarch should be applied to a stage III decubitus ulcer. ?

12. T   Adequate nutrition and fluid intake are required for healthy skin.

13. T   ferida
Bed sore is another term for decubitus ulcer.

14. F   If you think a change in a resident's skin isn't serious, then you don't need to report it.

15. T   força de cisalhamento
Shearing force can occur when you slide a resident across their bed.

ACTIVITY 3 - MATCHING

Match the nurse assistant's task with the preventative strategy.

Condition	Preventative Strategy
1. _D_ Helping an immobile resident maintain good circulation.	A. Mobility
2. _C_ Being attentive to any changes in the resident's skin condition.	B. Nutrition
3. _B_ Encouraging a resident to eat their meals.	C. Observation
4. _E_ Helping an incontinent resident to stay clean and dry.	D. Range-of-motion (ROM) exercise
5. _A_ Assisting a resident to ambulate.	E. Bathing/moisturizing
6. _F_ Telling the charge nurse about changes to a resident's skin.	F. Reporting

ACTIVITY 4 - MULTIPLE CHOICE

Circle the letter beside the best answer.

1. Skin that has integrity is:
   A. Tanned, tough, and thick.
   B. Free of moles or birth marks.
   C. Free of cuts, bruises, or wounds.
   D. Only found on babies and children.

2. What is a decubitus ulcer?
   A. A stomach ulcer that is caused by stress.
   B. An ulcer appearing only in people with AIDS.
   C. A wound that appears in pressure areas of the skin.
   D. An ulcer of the lips or mouth that is caused by a virus.

3. Shearing occurs when:
   A. You tear a sheet as you are making a bed.
   B. You put too much alcohol on a razor burn.
   C. Skin rubs against an object or another area of skin.
   D. A resident's skin remains damp for hours at a time.

4. Circulation of blood to the skin is enhanced by:
   A. Eating.
   B. Talking.
   C. Walking.
   D. Sleeping.

5. You can help maintain a resident's skin by:
   A. Inspecting it carefully every day.
   B. Taking them outside on sunny days.
   C. Giving them a daily dose of caster oil.
   D. Rubbing it hourly with antibiotic ointment.

ACTIVITY 5 – SITUATION/RESPONSE

Match the situation with the correct response.

Situation	Response
1. _____ Mrs. Leamus has thin, delicate skin. You notice that her thighs tend to stick to the toilet seat.	A. Encourage the resident to eat all their meals and drink plenty of fluids. Inspect the resident's skin daily. Be sure the bed linens are free of wrinkles before the resident goes to sleep.
2. _____ Mr. Mundt has a scratch on his elbow. It was caused by rough spot on the arm rest of his wheelchair.	B. Follow the charge nurse's instructions for treatment of the problem. Check frequently to see that the resident's heel is not resting on the bed.
3. _____ Mrs. Guillam is confined to bed. She is being treated for a stage II decubitus ulcer on her right heel.	C. Assist resident to the toilet on a frequent basis. When the resident wets themselves, clean their perineal area with soap and water before putting on a clean incontinence brief.
4. _____ Mrs. Crail is confused, underweight, and has little interest in food. When she sleeps, she tends to thrash around in bed, pulling at the sheets and covers.	D. Inspect the resident's thighs for skin breakdown. Use cornstarch on the toilet seat to prevent shearing. Notify the charge nurse about the situation.
5. _____ Mr. Karden is incontinent and wears an incontinence brief.	E. Ask the charge nurse what to do about the scratch. Place a pillow between the resident's arm and the arm rest until the rough spot can be removed from the arm rest.

ACTIVITY 6 – SKILLS PRACTICE

Using the Appendix Skills Checklists, practice the following skills:

Removing a Wound Dressing
Cleaning a Wound
Dressing a Wound

ACTIVITY 7 – LABELING

Label the following photos of decubitus ulcers correctly (Which is Stage I, II, III, or IV?)

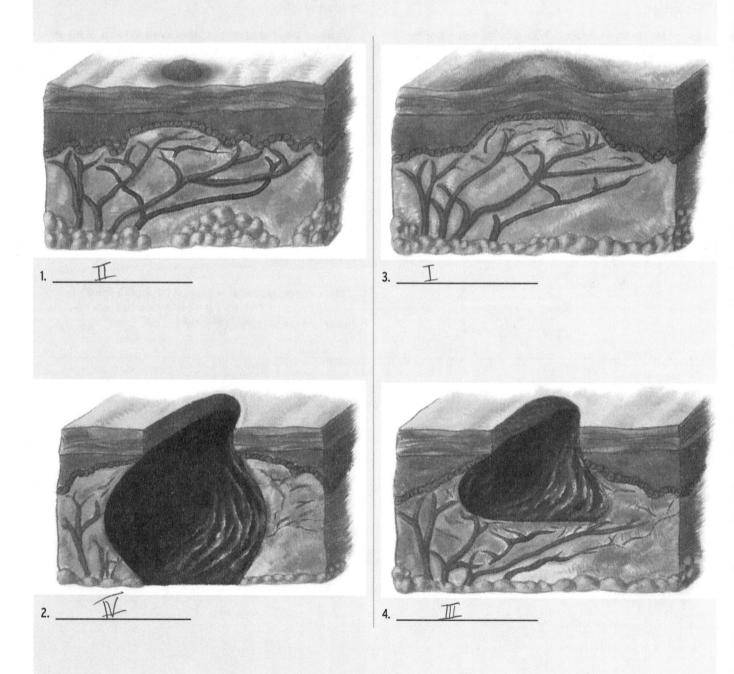

1. _____II_____

3. _____I_____

2. _____IV_____

4. _____III_____

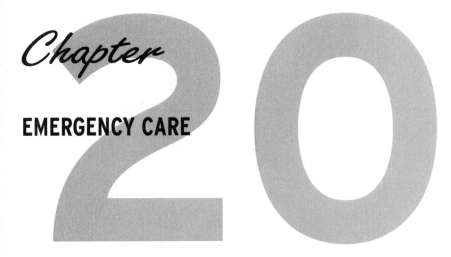

Chapter 20

EMERGENCY CARE

ACTIVITY 1 – MATCHING

In the space provided, write the letter of the description that defines the term.

Term	Definition
1. _E_ Aura	A. Excessive loss of blood in a short period of time.
2. _G_ Cardiopulmonary resuscitation (CPR)	B. Fatty deposits on blood vessel walls.
3. _B_ Cholesterol	C. Breastbone. _esterno_
4. _A_ Hemorrhage	D. A substance present in animal cells and body fluids.
5. _F_ Palpitations	E. A subtle sensation that often precedes a seizure.
6. _D_ Plaque	F. Strong, rapid heartbeats.
7. _H_ Protein	G. Procedure to maintain breathing and circulation in a person experiencing cardiac arrest.
8. _I_ Seizure _apreensão_	H. Combination of amino acids essential for all living cells.
9. _J_ Shock	I. A condition resulting from an abnormality in the brain.
10. _C_ Sternum	J. A condition in which vital organs in the body are not getting enough blood and oxygen to maintain good function.

ACTIVITY 2 – TRUE/FALSE

In the space provided, write T for true statements or F for false statements.

1. __F__ CPR should be performed on any unconscious resident.

2. __T__ Chest pain is a symptom of a seizure.

3. __T__ A person is hemorrhaging if they have lost 3 [1-2] quarts of blood.

4. __T__ Unusual thirst [punho] can be a symptom of shock.

5. __F__ The Heimlich maneuver is done to assist a person in cardiac arrest.

6. __F__ When one person does CPR, they should give two breaths for every 15 [2] [30] compressions.

7. __T__ Residents and visitors always know not to smoke in a room where oxygen is in use.

8. __T__ Heart attacks are caused by palpitations.

9. __T__ It is natural to feel nervous and scared during an emergency.

10. __T__ Cardiac arrest can result from a heart attack.

11. __T__ An airway obstruction causes a person to stop breathing.

12. __T__ Before having a seizure, a resident may feel an aura.

13. __F__ Electrical burns are caused by direct exposure to fire.

14. __T__ It's important to manage [gerir] your own feelings in an emergency.

15. __T__ When you give CPR, it's important to keep the victim's nose open at all times.

ACTIVITY 3 – LABELING

Using the word list, label the parts of the heart.

Word List

Right atrium
Valve (use twice)
Left atrium
Aorta
Left ventricle
Right ventricle

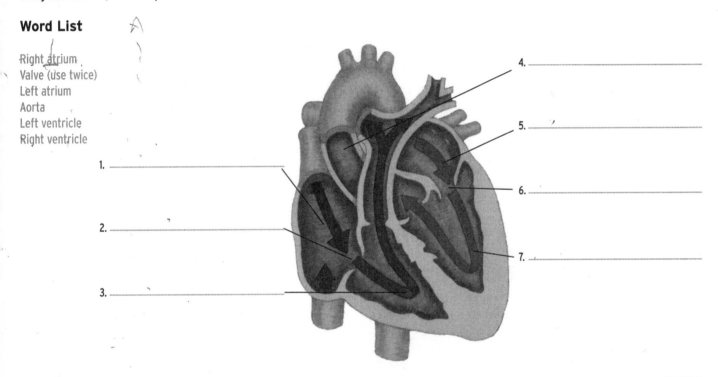

1. _____
2. _____
3. _____
4. _____
5. _____
6. _____
7. _____

ACTIVITY 4 – MULTIPLE CHOICE

Circle the letter next to the best answer.

1. In any emergency, a nurse assistant should stay with the resident, call for help, and:
   A. Remain calm.
   B. Always give first aid.
   C. Always give CPR.
   D. Take the resident's pulse.

2. You discover that a resident has a deep cut on their arm. What is the FIRST step you take?
   A. Put pressure on the wound.
   B. Call for the nurse.
   C. Have the resident lie down.
   D. Clean up any spilled blood.

3. Heart attacks are caused by:
   A. Difficulty breathing.
   B. Weakness and fatigue.
   C. A rapid, weak, irregular pulse.
   D. A blockage in the coronary arteries.

4. Cardiopulmonary resuscitation (CPR) is performed on a resident who:
   A. Is choking.
   B. Has cardiac arrest.
   C. Has cold and clammy skin.
   D. Does not respond to your touch.

5. What is one immediate treatment the charge nurse may ask you to do for a burn?
   A. Put butter or margarine on the burn.
   B. Run cold water over the burn.
   C. Put soap on the burn.
   D. Remove any jewelry that has stuck to the skin.

ACTIVITY 5 – LABELING

Using the descriptions provided, label each photo with the letter next to the correct description.

Photo Descriptions

A. Resident choking on food.
B. Nurse assistant giving the Heimlich maneuver to a resident.
C. Nurse assistant holding resident's hand under cool running water.
D. Nurse assistant opening a resident's airway.
E. Nurse assistant applying pressure to a bandage.
F. Nurse assistant giving artificial breaths to a mannequin.

1. E

4. A

2. D

5. B

3. F

6. C

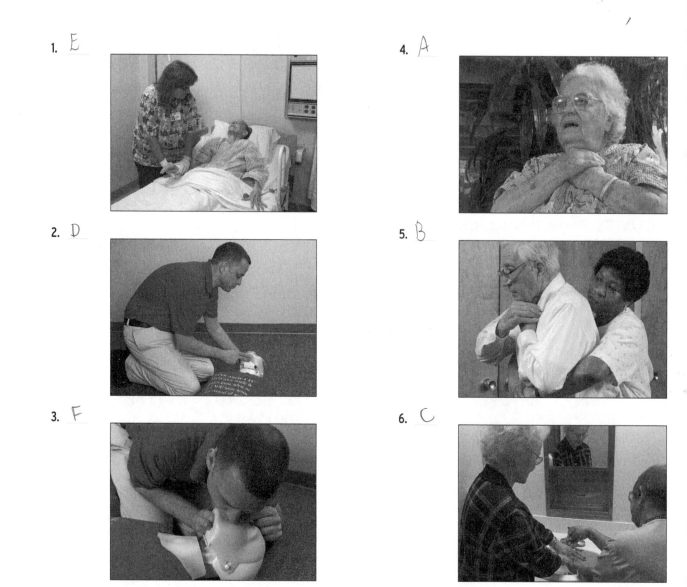

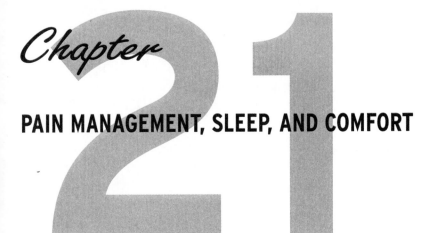

Chapter 21

PAIN MANAGEMENT, SLEEP, AND COMFORT

Using the definitions and clues provided, finish spelling out each word.

Acupuncture 4
Distraction 3
Endorphins 1

Guided imagery 5
Pain 2

1. These are natural morphine-like substances released by the brain during exercise, which can alter pain sensation:
   __ __ D __ __ __ __ __ N __

2. A bodily sensation that causes suffering and distress: __ __ __ N

3. This technique is used to direct a person's attention away from their pain or discomfort: __ __ __ T __ __ __ __ __ __ N

4. This is a medical therapy that originated in ancient China: __ C __ __ __ __ __ __ T __ __ __

5. Relaxation can be achieved through this technique involving words and music: __ U __ __ __ __ __ I __ __ __ __ __ R __

ACTIVITY 2 – TRUE/FALSE

Read each statement. In the space provided, write T if the statement is true and F if the statement is false.

1. __T__ Untreated pain can cause a decline in a resident's health.

2. __T__ A nurse assistant has an important role in helping a resident who has pain.

3. __T__ Most types of pain are a normal part of aging.

4. __F__ If a resident can smile, they are not in pain.

5. __T__ _ñ gerenciada._ Unmanaged pain can cause a person to feel depressed, anxious, and _temeroso_ fearful.

6. __T__ Hot applications are used to reduce swelling 24 hours after an injury.

7. __T__ Cold applications can help to control bleeding. _first 48 hours after a bruise or sprain immediately after some surgeries_

8. __T__ Unpleasant odors can prevent a resident from sleeping.

9. __T__ Pain is the fifth vital sign.

10. __T__ Residents have a right to have their pain treated.

ACTIVITY 3 – MATCHING

Match the misconception about pain with the fact.

Misconception	Fact
1. _____ It is better not to take pain medicine until the pain is really bad.	A. People can develop a tolerance to medication. It does not mean they are addicted or immune. They just need a stronger dose or a new medication.
2. _____ It is easier to deal with pain than the side effects of pain medication.	B. The risk of addiction is rare when the medication is taken for pain.
3. _____ If a resident takes too much pain medication, they will become addicted.	C. If you wait too long to take pain medicine, you may need a higher dose or stronger medicine. Taking medicine regularly can help prevent pain.
4. _____ Pain is a normal part of aging.	D. Pain happens more frequently for older people, but it is not normal and should be treated.
5. _____ If pain medicine no longer works for a resident, they must be addicted or immune to it.	E. It is important to treat pain. The nursing staff wants to help a resident who is in pain.
6. _____ Nurses and nurse assistants are too busy to be bothered about a resident's pain.	F. Pain medicines can cause side effects, but the side effects are treatable. Worries about side effects should not stop someone from taking pain medicine.

Dry heat= warm application

ACTIVITY 4 – MULTIPLE CHOICE

Circle the letter of the best answer.

1. What is the nurse assistant's role in helping residents who are in pain?
   A. To always offer the resident a hot compress for their pain.
   B. To always lead a resident through a guided imagery exercise.
   C. To always tell the charge nurse whenever a resident is in pain.
   D. To always notify the family whenever their loved one is in pain.

2. If a resident tells you their pain is a 3 on a scale of 10, what should you do?
   A. You should offer them an aspirin.
   B. You should tell the charge nurse promptly.
   C. You shouldn't do anything for so little pain.
   D. You should tell them not to worry until it is 8 or 9.

3. Untreated pain can cause a resident to feel:
   A. Sleepy.
   B. Hungry.
   C. Healthy.
   D. Hopeless.

banho de assento
4. A sitz bath is a type of:
   A. Dry cold.
   B. Moist heat.
   C. Acupuncture.
   D. Guided imagery.

efeito colateral
5. What is a common side effect of pain medication?
   A. Swelling.
   B. Itchy skin. *coceira*
   C. Incontinence.
   D. Constipation.

ACTIVITY 5 – MATCHING

Match the letter of the correct description to the non-drug therapy.

Non-drug therapy	Description
1. F Acupuncture	A. A technique that uses words and sometimes music to achieve a relaxed and focused state.
2. D Animals	B. Strategies to reduce anxiety, muscle tension, and pain that include meditation and deep breathing.
3. I Distraction	C. Laughter is used as a form of distraction.
4. A Guided imagery	D. Pet therapy programs provide relaxation and companionship as a form of distraction.
5. G Heat/cold application	E. A form of electrical massage applied to specific areas of the body.
6. C Humor	F. A *cura* healing method in which fine *agulhas* needles are inserted in the body at certain sites.
7. H Massage	G. This application is used in various dry or *umido* moist forms to relieve pain or increase comfort.
8. B Relaxation	H. A form of relaxation that involves the use of slow rhythmic strokes on specific areas of the body.
9. E Vibration	I. Technique in which the goal is to focus the resident's attention on something other than their pain.

Match each situation with the action a nurse assistant should take.

Situation	Response
1. ____ The charge nurse has applied a hot water bottle to a resident's hip to relieve pain.	A. Let the charge nurse know. It may be necessary for the resident to receive a laxative or stool softener.
2. ____ You notice Mrs. Carlton is rubbing her shoulder and grimacing. You ask her if she is in pain and she says "No."	B. Assure her that the nurse wants to know whenever a resident is in pain. Tell the charge nurse about the resident's pain.
3. ____ You notice that a resident seems to be in pain. You ask her about it, but she says she doesn't want to bother the nurse for medication.	C. Tell the charge nurse what you've observed and what the resident told you.
4. ____ You notice that a resident who is on pain medication has not had a bowel movement in two days.	D. Tell the charge nurse what you've noticed. Extra sleep may be a sign of over-medication.
5. ____ Mr. Acton has been on pain medication for three days. He has begun to sleep for several hours in the afternoon.	E. Follow the charge nurse's instructions. Check with the resident every 5 to 10 minutes. Check the site for signs of redness.

Refer to the textbook as needed to complete each exercise or answer each question.

1. Describe your own family's values concerning pain.

2. Should residents be expected to tolerate pain? Why or why not?

3. List three reasons a resident might try to hide their pain:

4. What is your most important responsibility for helping residents who are in pain?

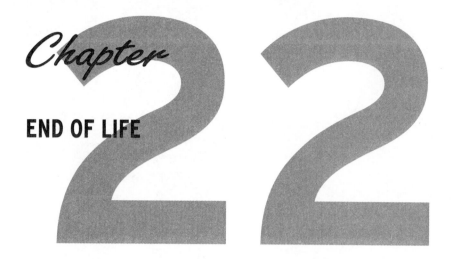

END OF LIFE

ACTIVITY 1 – MATCHING

Write the letter of the correct definition in the space provided by each term.

Term	Definition
1. _D_ Bereavement _D_	A. Care focused on comfort and symptom relief rather than cure
2. _C_ Hospice _C_	B. Rebirth in another form of life
3. _E_ Living will/advanced directive _E_	C. A program with a specially trained interdisciplinary team that cares for a terminally ill resident expected to die within six months
4. _A_ Palliative _A_	D. Period of grief after a loved one dies
5. _B_ Reincarnation _B_	E. A legal document used by a resident to communicate their wishes about the care they want if they become incapacitated and cannot make decisions
6. _F_ Postmortem _F_	F. After death

ACTIVITY 2 – MULTIPLE CHOICE

Circle the letter next to the best answer.

1. You can help a dying resident cope with their feelings by:
   A. Avoiding painful topics.
   B. Forcing them to face reality.
   C. Sharing your own views about death.
   D. Listening to anything they have to say.

2. What is an advance directive? *Living will*
   A. A last will and testament that is signed before the age of 50.
   B. A signed document which outlines a person's plan for reincarnation.
   C. A legal document stating the person's wishes about lifesaving care or death.
   D. A legal document stating what is to be done with your belongings after your death.

3. When a dying resident voices their anger, what should you say?
   A. "You shouldn't feel that way."
   B. "Everybody goes through this stage."
   C. "What you're going through is really hard, isn't it?"
   D. "Would you please try not to take your anger out on me?"

4. You can help the family of a dying resident by:
   A. Insisting that they pray with you.
   B. Telling them jokes or amusing stories.
   C. Helping them to laugh about their troubles.
   D. Being available to listen when they want to talk.

5. When a resident wants to talk about their funeral arrangements, it usually means they've reached the stage of:
   A. Resolution.
   B. Bargaining.
   C. Depression.
   D. Acceptance.

ACTIVITY 3 – TRUE/FALSE

In the space provided, write T if you think the statement is true or F if you think the statement is false.

1. **F** Everyone believes in life after death.

2. **T** Many people fear death because they are afraid of the unknown.

3. **F** The first stage of grief is bargaining.

4. **F** We all go through the stages of grief in an orderly progression.

5. **T** Bereavement is a period of grief someone goes through after a loved one dies.

6. **T** End of life care is the same as palliative care.

7. **T** Medicare covers hospice care for people who will die within 6 months.

8. **F** By forcing them to face reality, you help a dying resident reach acceptance.

9. **T** Reflection is a communication technique that may help a resident to talk about their feelings.

10. **F** The statement "I want to see my grandson graduate college," is an example of denial.

11. **T** If a dying resident seems unhappy with everything you do, they may be in the stage of anger.

12. **T** Family members of a dying resident always lose control of their emotions.

13. **F** It's OK to gossip about a resident after they have passed away.

14. **T** Just before death, a resident's eyes may stare blankly into space, with no eye movement.

15. **F** A resident's dentures should be discarded after death.

ACTIVITY 4 – SITUATION/RESPONSE

Read each situation. Write the letter of the appropriate response in the space provided.

Situation	Response
1. _____ Mrs. Littleton's roommate is very close to death. Mrs. Littleton seems agitated and upset, but doesn't seem willing to talk about her feelings.	A. Let the charge nurse know what you've observed. She may choose to talk with the resident's daughter about the stages of grief. The resident seems to be in denial.
2. _____ Mrs. Jackson is visiting her mother, who has been lingering close to death for a week. Mrs. Jackson has lost control of her emotions and is crying uncontrollably.	B. Respect her beliefs about reincarnation. Listen attentively when she talks, but don't force a discussion about your viewpoint.
3. _____ Mr. Montgomery has recently been told his lung cancer has spread to his liver and stomach. He has never seemed more cheerful. When his daughter tries to talk to him about signing an advance directive, he becomes angry and changes the subject.	C. Share your feelings with a trusted co-worker or friend. Remember that this is an awkward and painful time for the family. They may not ever thank you for all you have done for their loved one. You may have to comfort yourself by remembering the nice times you shared with the resident.
4. _____ Mrs. Spencer tells you that in a previous life she was a spiritual healer for a tribe of ancient Indians. You think this is ridiculous.	D. Give her an opportunity to open up about her feelings. Say something like, "You and your roommate have been such good friends; you must be very sad right now." If she doesn't want to talk, don't try to make her do so.
5. _____ One of your favorite residents is very close to death. You have been an important person in her life for over two years, but the family is ignoring you during these final hours. Your feelings are hurt.	E. Guide her to a private or secluded area. Offer her a tissue. Pay attention to her non-verbal communication. If she seems to want privacy, leave her alone. If she wants you to stay, begin a conversation with a statement like, "This must be very difficult for you."

ACTIVITY 5 – QUESTIONS TO CONSIDER

1. Do you have any fears about death? What helps you manage these fears?

_____

_____

_____

_____

2. Have you had anyone close to you die? What did you feel when you learned about their death?

_____

_____

_____

_____

3. What religious or other rituals were a part of your saying goodbye to your loved one? How did these rituals help?

_____

_____

_____

_____

4. What are some ways you can assist the dying resident's family during the process of dying?

_____

_____

_____

_____

5. List some ways you can assist residents in coping with the death of another resident. What may be their major concerns?

_____

_____

_____

_____

6. How will you deal with residents dying? List ways you can cope.

_____

_____

_____

_____

Chapter

23

OTHER WORK ENVIRONMENTS AND RESIDENT POPULATIONS

ACTIVITY 1 – FILL IN THE BLANK

Using the list of terms, complete each sentence correctly.

3 Agenda behavior   9 Behavioral symptoms   11 Hallucination   *vagando* (Wandering)
4 Agitation   10 Cognitive impairment   8 Insomnia
2 Alzheimer's disease   1 Delusion *(ilusão)*   13 Multi-infarct
12 Anxiety   Dementia   7 Sundown syndrome
                         5

1. A false <u>thought</u> *(pensamento)* that is thought to be real is called a(n) _____.

2. _____ _____ is a progressive, incurable disease that affects the brain and causes memory loss and eventual death.

3. When a resident tends to follow a certain agenda, often a past routine, their behavior is referred to as _____ _____.

4. A resident's movements that are irregular, rapid, violent, or excited and often troubled suggest the resident is experiencing

   _____.

5. Actions that are caused by a disease or condition are known as _____.

6. When a person moves from one place to another <u>aimlessly</u> *(sem rumo)*, they are _____.

7. _____ _____ is a situation later in the day when a resident may become irritable or combative, or tearful and withdrawn.

8. When a person cannot sleep enough, they have _____.

9. _____ means that a person is experiencing a disruption in knowledge, memory, awareness, or judgment.

10. The term _____ refers to a loss of mental functions such as memory, thinking, and reasoning.

11. A person is having a(n) _____ when they see or hear things that are not really there.

12. _____ is a state of <u>uneasiness</u> *(inquietação)* in the mind.

13. _____ - _____ is a type of damage to blood vessels that may cause a loss of function in a tissue or organ, such as the brain.

ACTIVITY 2 – SPELL IT OUT

Using the clues and terms provided, complete the spelling of each word.

2 Confront   5 Distraction   1 Maximize   4 Technique   3 Validation

1. To increase something to the maximum: ___ ___ ___ ___ M ___ ___ ___

2. To face someone with a challenge: ___ ___ ___ F ___ ___ ___ ___

3. Confirmation of something: ___ ___ ___ ___ D ___ ___ ___ N

4. A method for reaching a desired goal: ___ ___ C ___ ___ ___ ___ ___ E

5. Something that distracts the resident's attention or eases mental confusion: ___ ___ S ___ R ___ ___ ___ ___ ___ ___

ACTIVITY 3 – MULTIPLE CHOICE

Circle the best answer to each question.

1. Alzheimer's disease is a form of:
    A. Cancer.
    X Dementia.
    C. Osteoporosis.
    D. Cerebral palsy.

2. How can you prevent a resident who has dementia from becoming agitated?
    A. Confine the resident to their room.
    X Provide a quiet, controlled environment.
    C. Repeatedly tell the resident to stay calm.
    D. Provide lots of exciting large group activities.

3. Mrs. Dodson says everyone wants to steal her things. This suggests she is:
    X Delusional. _delirante_
    B. Short of breath. _falta de ar_
    C. Hard of hearing.
    D. Just teasing the staff.

4. One of your responsibilities in caring for residents with dementia is to:
    X Anticipate their basic needs.
    B. Give them presents on holidays.
    C. Hide _ocultar_ them from family members.
    D. Prevent them from taking too much of your time.

5. Mr. Smith tells you he has to go to work today. Using the technique called validation therapy, how would you respond to his demand to go to work?
    A. Tell him that he is too old and sick to work.
    B. Ignore his continued requests for your attention.
    X Tell him today is a holiday and he doesn't have to work.
    D. Remind him that he is retired and has Alzheimer's disease.

Match each behavioral term with the example of that behavior and an approach to care.

1. _____ Mr. Alvin doesn't do crossword puzzles anymore and always seems sad and tired. You encourage him to talk about how he feels.

2. _____ Mr. Hendricks taps his foot on the floor repeatedly. You make sure there is no physical problem causing his distress.

3. _____ Mrs. Penrose has an increased pulse rate and appears tense. You assure her that she is safe.

4. _____ Mrs. Rushman never sleeps more than two hours a night. You help her to eat properly and rest during the day.

5. _____ Mrs. Wiley believes that her family wants to hurt her. You help her feel loved and supported, without arguing about her beliefs.

6. _____ Mr. Randall sometimes has conversations with people who are not there. You listen to him without questioning who he is talking to.

7. _____ Mr. Williamson walks up and down the hallway, opening and closing doors. You help him get routine exercise.

A. Agitation

B. Anxiety

C. Delusions

D. Depression

E. Hallucinations

F. Insomnia

G. Wandering

ACTIVITY 5 – RESPONSIBILITY REVIEW

List the six principles that guide your activities when caring for residents with Alzheimer's disease. Refer to your textbook as needed to complete this exercise. Hint: one principle is to "Provide Guidance and Direction."

1a. _____

2a. _____

3a. _____

4a. _____

5a. _____

6a. _____

List the six techniques that will help you support the resident and lessen the intensity of some behavioral symptoms. Refer to your textbook as needed to complete this exercise. Hint: one technique is to "Enter a Resident's Reality."

1b. _____

2b. _____

3b. _____

4b _____

5b. _____

6b. _____

ACTIVITY 6 – MATCHING

Match the factors that cause resistance to care with the description of that factor.

Factor	Description
1. _B_ Medical/emotional factors	A. Responding to your negative body language, tone of voice, or facial expressions.
2. _A_ Communication factors	B. <ins>ñ satisfazer</ins> <ins>Unmet</ins> basic needs such as hunger, thirst, pain or the need for elimination.
3. _E_ Environmental factors	C. The resident's needs change as the disease progresses.
4. _D_ Nature of the task	D. The resident may not understand the procedure or what is expected of them.
5. _C_ Stage of the disease	E. The room may be too cold, too dark, have too much equipment, etc.

ACTIVITY 7 – STRATEGY REVIEW

Describe a strategy you can use to overcome resistance caused by each of these factors listed in Activity 6.

1. Medical/emotional factors:

   _____

   _____

2. Communication factors:

   _____

   _____

3. Environmental factors:

   _____

   _____

4. Nature of the task:

   _____

   _____

5. Stage of the disease:

   _____

   _____

ACTIVITY 8 – CONTENT REVIEW

For each activity of daily living listed below, write two guidelines you can use to assist a resident who has dementia. Refer to your textbook as needed to complete this exercise.

Toileting

1. _____

2. _____

Hydration

3. _____

4. _____

Eating

5 _____

6. _____

Dressing

7. _____

8. _____

Bathing

9. _____

10. _____

Grooming

11. _____

12. _____

ACTIVITY 9 – QUESTION & ANSWER

Refer to the textbook as needed to complete each exercise or answer each question.

1. Have you ever thought to yourself, "I can't absorb any more information. My head is spinning"? What do you do in situations like this?

2. What do you think it is like to feel overwhelmed every moment of your life?

3. How would you want the people around you to behave when you are feeling overwhelmed?

ACTIVITY 10 - FILL IN THE BLANK

Using the terms provided below, complete each sentence correctly.

7 Adaptive skills   8 Developmental disability   1 Habilitation model   10 Mental retardation
2 Autism   9 Down syndrome   4 Individual service plan   11 Normalization
3 Cerebral palsy   5 Epilepsy   6 IQ test

1. A philosophy of care in which an individual with a developmental disability is educated or trained to participate as fully as possible in all aspects of life, including interaction with their family and community, and to have a satisfying social life, is called the

   _____ _____ .

2. _____ is a disorder in which the child withdraws from the world; the cause is not known, and there is no cure.

3. Damage to the central nervous system before, during, or after birth can cause _____ _____ .

4. An individual program plan, also known as _____ _____ _____ , is a plan of care that provides special accommodations and sets the priorities of care for the resident.

5. _____ is a disorder of the nervous system that causes seizures and may cause a developmental disability.

6. A(n) _____ is a measure of a person's intelligence.

7. People use _____ _____ everyday to live, work, and play.

8. A(n) _____ _____ is a chronic, severe condition that a person develops from any of many causes, which prevents them from living independently without assistance.

9. _____ _____ is a condition in which a person is born with an extra chromosome, causing some level of mental retardation, abnormal features, and often other medical problems; also known as mongolism and trisomy 21 syndrome.

10. An individual has _____ _____ *abaixo da media* when they have significantly below-average intelligence and minimal adaptive skills.

11. The creation of an environment for individuals with developmental disabilities that is as close to normal as possible is called

    _____ .

ACTIVITY 11 – MULTIPLE CHOICE

Circle the letter of the best answer.

1. Assisted living facilities are also known as:
   A. Subacute care facilities.
   B. Residential care facilities.
   C. Inpatient recovery centers.
   D. Radiation treatment centers.

2. What is a typical example of a person in a subacute care unit?
   A. A person who has mental retardation.
   B. A person suffering from chicken pox or measles.
   C. A person with a severe developmental disability.
   D. A person who has had knee replacement surgery.

3. Which of these conditions is always present before birth?
   A. Autism.
   B. Epilepsy.
   C. Down syndrome.
   D. Mental retardation.

4. What is fragile X syndrome?
   A. A mild infection.
   B. A genetic disorder.
   C. Fetal alcohol syndrome.
   D. A virus that causes fragile bones.

5. What is another name for an individual habilitation plan?
   A. Annual progress report.
   B. Individual program plan.
   C. Interdisciplinary care plan.
   D. Normalization status report.

ACTIVITY 12 – TRUE/FALSE

In the space provided, write T for true or F for false.

1. __T__ Autism varies from person to person.

2. __T__ Most people use their adaptive skills everyday.

3. __T__ The typical stay in a subacute care facility is less than 30 days.

4. __F__ Residents in assisted living facilities must cook their own meals.

5. __T__ The abbreviation "IQ" means intelligence quotient.

6. __F__ People with epilepsy are rarely able to hold jobs.

7. __T__ Cerebral palsy can occur after birth.

8. __F__ A person who has Down syndrome is missing an extremity.

9. __F__ You can always tell a person has HIV by the way they look.

10. __T__ Facilities that care for intellectually/developmentally disabled persons are called ICF/MR facilities.

ACTIVITY 13 – CONTENT REVIEW

Read each description below. In the space provided, write the name of the disease or disability that applies.

Autism
Cerebral palsy
Down syndrome
Epilepsy
HIV/AIDS
Mental retardation

Mr. Wilkins is 28 years old and lives in a group home. He is short and his face is noticeable because of his slanted eyes and protruding tongue. He is able to communicate, bathe, dress, and feed himself. He is not able to hold a job or attend a regular school.

1. _____

Betsy is 10 years old and has frequent convulsions. She is on medication to control the convulsions, but must live in a facility where her condition can be controlled. She attends a special school.

2. _____

Teddy is 8 years old, and has a normal appearance. He does not respond to the people around him and does not liked to be touched. He sometimes bangs his head against the wall and chants words or phrases over and over. He lives in a group home and requires constant supervision.

3. _____

Mr. Dickenson is 36 years old and lives in a group home. He lacks the intelligence needed to take care of his basic needs. He cannot leave the facility without supervision and assistance.

4. _____

Janie is 14 years old and lives in a facility for the developmentally disabled. She has mild paralysis in her arms and legs and spends her days in a special wheelchair. She talks with great difficulty and sometimes has seizures. She receives ROM exercises daily.

5. _____

Mr. Russo is a former drug abuser who lives in a nursing facility. He is underweight and suffers from skin rashes, diarrhea, and fatigue. He frequently has a fever. His disease has no cure.

6. _____

ACTIVITY 14 – CRITICAL THINKING

1. Think about working in the settings that have been described in this chapter. Based on what you have learned, describe how caregiving would be different in each of these types of facilities. How would you adapt your care?

Assisted Living Facility

_____

_____

_____

Subacute Care Unit

_____

_____

_____

ICF/MR

_____

_____

_____

HIV/AIDS Unit

_____

_____

_____

Chapter
24
SPECIALTY SKILLS FOR SUBACUTE ENVIRONMENTS

ACTIVITY 1 – FILL IN THE BLANK

Complete each sentence by adding the correct term.

6 Artificial airway	10 Dialysis	7 Endotracheal tube	9 Hemodialysis
8 Blood sugar	4 Diaphragmatic breathing	3 Enteral nutrition	2 Hyperglycemia
5 Cold Compress	11 Dry heat	1 Fasting blood sugar	

1. _____ is a test of blood glucose level using a blood sample (from a prick in a finger or ear or through a needle from a vein) taken at least eight hours after last eating.

2. Blood sugar level that is too high is known as _____.

3. Providing liquid nourishment through a tube passed into the nose and down to the stomach (a nasogastric tube, or NGT) or a tube surgically inserted through the abdominal wall into the stomach (a gastrostomy tube, or G-tube) is called _____.

4. Deep breathing that uses muscles of the abdomen is known as _____.

5. A(n) _____ is a dry cold application.

6. A tube placed through the mouth or nose into the trachea for breathing is a(n) _____.

7. A(n) _____ is a tube placed into the trachea of a person's respiratory system, through the nose, mouth, or surgically through a stoma in the neck, to assist in breathing.

8. _____ measures the amount of one type of sugar (glucose) in the blood.

9. A process for removing waste and fluid directly from the person's blood through a tube that has been surgically implanted; the tube is connected to an artificial kidney machine that filters and returns the blood to the person is known as _____.

10. _____ is a method used to artificially remove waste from the blood when the kidneys are not functioning well.

11. A dry warm application is called _____.

ACTIVITY 2 – MATCHING

In the space provided, write the letter of the description that defines the term.

1. __E__ Nasal cannula

2. __B__ Sitz bath

3. __C__ Oxygen

4. __A__ Moist heat

5. __F__ Oropharyngeal tube

6. __I__ Total parenteral nutrition

7. __D__ Incentive spirometer

8. __M__ Moist cold

9. __G__ Hypoglycemia

10. __J__ Tracheostomy tube

11. __H__ Peritoneal dialysis

12. __N__ Mechanical ventilator

13. __K__ Tracheostomy

14. __L__ Hypoxia

A. Moist warm application.

B. A bath in a tub or special basin in which only the perineum and buttocks are immersed.

C. An odorless, tasteless, and colorless gas.

D. A device that measures and shows how deeply a person breathes, seeing the result helps to encourage deep breathing.

E. Two-pronged tube inserted into the nostrils *narinas* to deliver oxygen.

F. A tube placed through the mouth into the pharynx *faringe* for breathing.

G. Blood sugar level that is too low.

H. Process used for removing waste and fluid from the blood through a surgically placed catheter in the abdominal (peritoneal) cavity.

I. Nutrition administered intravenously.

J. A breathing tube placed directly into the trachea through a surgical opening (stoma) in the person's neck.

K. A stoma through the trachea into the respiratory airway.

L. A state in which the blood oxygen level shows that the body is not getting enough oxygen.

M. Moist cold application.

N. A machine used to assist or replace spontaneous breathing when a person cannot breathe on their own.

ACTIVITY 3 – TRUE/FALSE

In the space provided, write T for true or F for false.

1. __T__ Heat or cold may be applied to the entire body for a general effect.

2. __F__ Heat stops tissue from healing. _cura_

3. __F__ People who are on a subacute floor usually need care for a long time.

4. __F__ Fasting blood sugars are taken after someone eats.

5. __T__ Diaphragmatic breathing is deep breathing that uses the muscles of the abdomen rather than the chest muscles.

6. __T__ Some residents may breathe easier if positioned on one side or another.

7. __F__ Postural drainage involves walking the resident every four hours.

8. __F__ Hypoxia helps a person.

9. __T__ Oxygen is an odorless, tasteless, and colorless gas.

10. __T__ It is important to inspect the inside of shoes for foreign objects or areas of roughness if the person has diabetes.

ACTIVITY 4 – SKILLS PRACTICE

Using the Appendix Skills Checklists, practice the following skills:

Blood Glucose Monitoring by Finger Prick
Diabetic Foot Care
Assisting With Diaphragmatic Breathing
Assisting With Deep Breathing and Coughing
Assisting With Incentive Spirometer
Administering Oxygen by Nasal Cannula
Administering Oxygen by Simple Face Mask

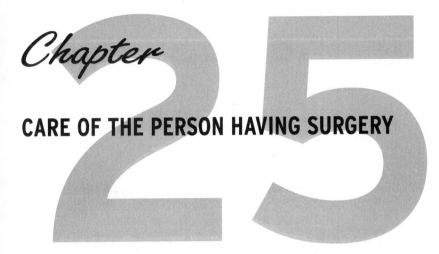

CARE OF THE PERSON HAVING SURGERY

ACTIVITY 1 – FILL IN THE BLANK

Using the medical terms below, complete each sentence.

Anesthesia 3
Anesthetic 7
Anti-embolism stockings 8

Emesis basin 5
Postoperative 6
Preoperative 2

Prosthesis 4
Splint 1

1. A(n) _____ is used to hold or keep an area from moving.

2. The time before surgery is called _____.

3. A state of being unaware or unable to feel is called _____.

4. A device that substitutes and functions in the place of a missing body part is called a(n) _____.

5. A(n) _____ is a special basin used to catch vomit or secretions coughed up.

6. The time after surgery is called _____.

7. _____ is the medication given to a person before surgery.

8. _____ are often worn after surgery to help prevent blood clots.

ACTIVITY 2 - YES OR NO?

Beside each example, write YES if it would be a fear and NO if it would not be a fear.

1. _____ Will I be unconscious for a long time?

2. _____ Will I look different after surgery?

3. _____ When can I have visitors after the surgery?

4. _____ Will I get ice cream after my surgery?

5. _____ Is the surgeon good looking?

6. _____ Are there any complication with this surgery?

7. _____ How long will the surgery take?

8. _____ What if I don't wake up from the anesthesia?

9. _____ Are there a lot of risks with this surgery?

10. _____ Will I have a big scar from the surgery?

ACTIVITY 3 - TRUE OR FALSE

Write T for True or F for False next to each example.

1. _____ Patients need to remove all jewelry before surgery.

2. _____ A surgical consent form needs to be filled out.

3. _____ An ID bracelet with the correct information is put on the person's wrist.

4. _____ The patient can wear their wig during surgery.

5. _____ The nurse who gives the medications records the name of the medication, the dose, the route and the time administered.

6. _____ Nail polish can be worn during surgery.

7. _____ The recovery room staff calls ahead to alert staff that the person is ready to be moved from the recovery room.

8. _____ Any known allergies should be reported.

9 _____ A lab report may include the person's blood type.

10. _____ A surgical admission sheet would include the family's telephone numbers.

ACTIVITY 4 - SKILLS PRACTICE

Using the Appendix Skills Checklists, practice the following skills:

Shaving the Surgical Site
Assisting With Deep Breathing and Coughing

ACTIVITY 5 – INTERVIEWING SKILLS

Using the pre-op checklist find a classmate or family member who you can interview to complete the pre-op checklist below.

PRE-OP CHECK LIST
DEPARTMENT OF NURSING

Check List
This list must accompany each patient
Nurse preparing the patient must complete and sign checklist form
Nurse releasing the patient must verify the patient's id and sign form
List to be kept with patient's record until discharged then destroyed

Identification Bands		**Clinical data in chart** ( )	
A) Arm ( )		CBC	EKG if ordered
B) Leg ( )		Urinalysis	Blood set up as ordered
C) Allergy ( )		Chest X-ray	
Skin Preparations ( )		Medication charted ( )	
Note abnormalities		Medication sheet sent w/patient ( )	
Vital signs recorded ( )		**Record assembled** ( )	
Height and weight ( )		Current record	Medication sheet
Catheterized ( )		Old records	Vital signs sheets
Voided ( )		X-ray	Doctor's order sheet
Time _____		Other	
Amount _____			
Dress		Pre op orders reviewed ( )	
A) Hospital gown ( )		Procedure consent ( )	
B) Hair pins, wigs removed ( )		Anesthesia consent ( )	
C) Nail polish removed ( )			

Valuable checklist	none	removed	not removed
1. Dentures upper	( )	( )	( )
lower	( )	( )	( )
2. Glasses	( )	( )	( )
3. Contacts	( )	( )	( )
4. Prosthetic-devises	( )	( )	( )
5. Jewelry/earrings	( )	( )	( )
6. Hearing aids	( )	( )	( )
7. Other	( )	( )	( )

Chapter 26

SPECIAL SKILLS FOR SPECIAL TIMES

ACTIVITY 1 – FILL IN THE BLANK

Using the medical terms below, complete each sentence.

Amniotic sac 2   Epidural 5   Placenta 7
Cervix 4   Labor 1   Prenatal 8
Cesarean section 6   Neonate 3

1. Stages of expulsion of the fetus from the uterus through the vagina, beginning with contractions and the release of amniotic fluid and ending with delivery is called _____ .

2. _____ _____ is a membrane that encloses the fetus inside the uterus; it contains amniotic fluid that cushions and supports the fetus during development.

3. A newborn infant up to one month of age is known as a(n) _____ .

4. The _____ is an opening of the uterus into the vagina.

5. A(n) _____ is a type of anesthetic given by injection to minimize the pain of childbirth.

6. Giving birth through a surgical incision made through the abdomen into the uterus is known as a(n) _____

    _____ .

7. _____ is a temporary organ that develops in the uterus during pregnancy to transfer oxygen and nutrients to the fetus and remove carbon dioxide and some waste products: commonly called "the afterbirth."

8. _____ is the period of pregnancy before childbirth.

ACTIVITY 2 – SPELL IT OUT

Using the terms provided, spell out each word beside the correct description.

Colostrum 1   Express 7   Lactation 3   Trimester 2
Delivery   Fundus 6   Lochia 5
Engorgement 9   Immunization 8   Postpartum 4

1. The watery "first milk" that appears from a newborn mother's breasts is called _ _ _ _ O _ T _ _ _ _ .

2. One third of the normal period of pregnancy is called _ _ R _ _ _ _ _ _ R.

3. The production of breast milk is known as _ _ A _ T _ _ _ _ _ .

4. _ O _ _ P _ _ _ _ _ _ is the period after childbirth.

5. _ _ _ _ C _ _ A is a vaginal discharge that occurs after childbirth.

6. The top of the uterus is called _ _ _ N _ _ _ .

7. A technique used by a breastfeeding mother to remove breast milk to a container to be used later for bottle feeding is called _ _ _ P _ _ _ _ .

8. _ _ M _ N _ _ T _ _ _ _ _ means being protected against a disease by vaccination.

9. A postpartum mother's breast being swollen with milk is known as _ _ _ _ _ _ R _ _ M _ _ _ T.

ACTIVITY 3 – MATCHING

Match the letter next to each definition with the correct term for that definition.

1. B Circumcision

2. C Episiotomy

3. A Delivery

4. D Umbilical cord

A. The act of giving birth.

B. The surgical removal of the foreskin at the head of the penis.

C. A surgical incision made to enlarge the vaginal opening for child birth.

D. A tube connecting the fetus to the mother's placenta.

Name two signs and symptoms of a normal first trimester:

1. _____

2. _____

Name two signs and symptoms of a normal second trimester:

1. _____

2. _____

Name two signs and symptoms of a normal third trimester:

1. _____

2. _____

ACTIVITY 5 – SKILLS PRACTICE

Using the Appendix Skills Checklists, practice the following skills:

Assisting With a Sitz Bath
Diapering a Newborn
Bathing a Newborn
Care of a Circumcision

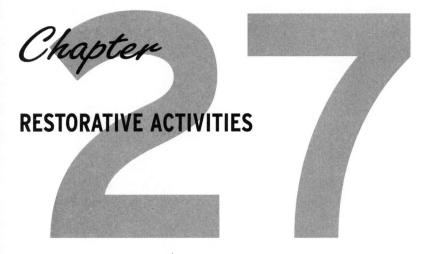

RESTORATIVE ACTIVITIES

ACTIVITY 1 – MATCHING

In the space provided, write the letter of the correct definition for each term.

1. _A_ **Brace** (braçadeira)   A. device that supports and strengthens a body part

2. _C_ **Extremity**   B. supportive equipment made for a resident, such as a _brace_ or _splint_ that supports a limb   braçadeira tala   membro

3. _B_ **Orthotic device**   C. a limb of the body

4. _D_ **Prosthetic device**   D. device made to replace a missing body part or function

5. _E_ **Rehabilitation**   E. the process of restoring to a former state

6. _H_ **Reinforce**   F. device to use to support or immobilize a body part

7. _I_ **Restorative**   G. a short horizontal bar suspended by two parallel ropes, used to pull oneself up in bed

8. _F_ **Splint** (tala)   H. to strengthen something

9. _G_ **Trapeze**   I. restore to a former state

ACTIVITY 2 – FILL IN THE BLANK

Using the terms provided below, complete each sentence correctly.

Alert   Function   Optimal
Artificial limb Immobilized   Prompting
Capability   Independence   Regain
Cuing   Maintain   Stump

1. The portion of an extremity remaining after the rest is removed is called the _____.

2. In order to keep something in its existing state, it is necessary to _____ it.

3. Restorative activities are done in a way to help restore _____, or the action for which a body part is used.

4. If someone is quick to perceive and act on a situation, they are _____.

5. When you give a resident a signal to begin a specific speech or action, you are _____.

6. Moving a person to take an action, or helping them remember something is called _____.

7. In order to prevent freedom of movement, a joint or body part must be _____.

8. The goal of restorative activities is to help a resident achieve their most desirable, or _____, level of functioning.

9. An arm or leg that is human-made is called a(n) _____ _____.

10. _____ refers to a person's ability to do something.

11. A person who is not subject to control by others has _____.

12. Restorative activities can help a person _____ lost function again.

ACTIVITY 3 – MULTIPLE CHOICE

Circle the letter beside the best answer.

1. You are working with a resident who recently had a stroke. It takes the resident a long time to dress himself. How can you help him regain lost function?
    A. Insist on doing everything for him.
    B. Tell the family to help him every day.
    C. Help him so that he gets dressed faster.
    D. Be patient and let him do as much as he can.

2. The nurse asks you to give range-of-motion exercise to Mrs. White, who is confined to bed. According to her care plan, there are no restrictions. What does "no restrictions" mean?
    A. You should work her joints and muscles very hard.
    B. Provide ROM exercise as often as possible on each shift.
    C. Mrs. White should be able to do all of the exercises herself.
    D. You may move each joint through its full available range.

3. Mrs. Wilson seems puzzled or confused when you tell her you'd like her to practice using a walker. How can you help her understand?
    A. Tell her you are in a hurry.
    B. Repeat the request in a different way.
    C. Use baby talk to get your point across.
    D. Tell the next shift nurse assistant to try it.

4. Which of the following is an orthotic device?
    A. Walker
    B. Trapeze
    C. Leg brace
    D. Artificial leg

5. You are about to help Mrs. Paulsen take a walk. She is on oxygen. What is the BEST way to ensure her safety?
    A. Have her take a few deep breaths before you walk.
    B. Carry her oxygen tank under your arm as you walk.
    C. Take her off oxygen for the short time she is walking.
    D. Ask another staff to follow and pull a portable oxygen tank.

ACTIVITY 4 – INDEPENDENT/DEPENDENT

Read the following sentences. In the space provided, write I if the action promotes independence or D if it promotes dependence.

1. _____ A resident wants to walk to the dining room, but you tell him you can get him there quicker by pushing him in a wheelchair.

2. _____ You give a resident a bed bath even though with assistance they could take a shower.

3. _____ You encourage a resident to take a walk while you make the bed.

4. _____ You wheel a resident to the activities room.

5. _____ You encourage a resident to use his cane to take a walk.

6. _____ You say to a resident, "I'll start buttoning your shirt, and you can finish it."

7. _____ A resident can walk a little, but you use a wheelchair all the time.

8. _____ A resident picks up a spoon to eat, but because they are slow you take the spoon and begin feeding them.

9. _____ You hand a piece of bread to a resident who is recovering from a stroke, encouraging them to use their weak hand.

10. _____ You discuss a resident's eating limitations with the charge nurse in hopes of coming up with some assistive devices so they can eat without your help.

ACTIVITY 5 – CONTENT REVIEW

List two examples in each category of equipment. Refer to your textbook if necessary.

Assistive devices

1. walker

2. Cane

Prosthetic and orthotic devices

1. Braces

2. artificial limb

Positioning devices

1. Pillows

2. Trapeze

Aids for activities of daily living

1. eye glasses

2. hearing aids

ACTIVITY 6 – TRUE/FALSE

Read the following sentences. In the space provided, write T if the statement is true or F if the statement is false.

1. _T_ A contracture occurs when a joint becomes stuck in a certain position.

2. _F_ Once the interdisciplinary team sets goals for a resident, those goals never change.

3. _F_ A disability is a physical problem only and never affects a resident's psychological state.

4. _F_ Prompting and cuing are forms of sign language used only to communicate with hearing impaired individuals.

5. _T_ One goal of restorative activities is to enable a resident to perform activities of daily living independently.

6. _F_ An entire ROM exercise program always takes about 60 minutes.

7. _T_ You perform finger flexion when you bend the fingers at each of the joints.

8. _T_ Each range of motion exercise should be repeated 5 to 10 times, depending on the resident's comfort level.

ACTIVITY 7 – SKILLS PRACTICE

Using the Appendix Skills Checklists, practice the following skills:

Range of Motion Exercises
Assisting With Walking

ACTIVITY 8 – CONTENT REVIEW

List two examples of short- and long-term goals the following residents undergoing rehabilitation might try to achieve. Refer to your textbook if necessary.

Resident 1

Mrs. Hildebrand is recovering from total hip replacement surgery. She is able to sit up on the side of the bed.

1. Short-term goal:

2. Long-term goal:

Resident 2

Mr. Scott recently had a leg amputated below the knee. He has just received his prosthetic leg and is receiving physical therapy each day.

3. Short-term goal:

4. Long-term goal:

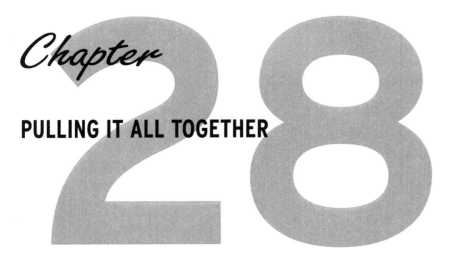

Chapter 28

PULLING IT ALL TOGETHER

ACTIVITY 1 – TRUE/FALSE

In the space provided, write T if you think the statement is true or F if you think the statement is false.

1. __T__ You treat residents as individuals when you give care based on their preferences.

2. __F__ "Prioritizing" means you should do the most difficult tasks last.

3. __F__ The charge nurse can help you learn how to organize your time.

4. __T__ You are mindful when you balance the skill and the art of caregiving.

5. __T__ One responsibility of the night shift is to prepare paperwork for the next day.

6. __F__ You should never do a task that is normally done on another shift.

7. __T__ The residents' needs determine which resident is cared for first.

8. __T__ Time management is a critical skill for a nurse assistant.

9. __F__ You must keep to a schedule _independente_ regardless of the needs of individual residents.

10. __T__ Making rounds before you begin specific tasks is important.

ACTIVITY 2 – MULTIPLE CHOICE

Circle the letter next to the best answer.

1. If you want to get along with residents and co-workers, you should always be:
   A. Content.
   B. Confusing.
   C. Considerate.
   D. Conservative.

2. How can you be a <u>mindful caregiver</u>?
   A. Consider the resident's preferences.
   B. Keep your residents on a consistent schedule.
   C. If a resident can't do a task quickly, do it for them.
   D. Never let a resident wear a dress twice in one week.

3. Using time management skills can help you <u>avoid:</u> _evitar_
   A. Feeling unhappy.
   B. Feeling nauseous.
   C. Feeling disorganized. _o_
   D. Feeling unappreciated.

4. How should you prioritize tasks?
   A. By the tasks that take the least time.
   B. By the tasks that need to be done soonest.
   C. By the tasks left over from the previous shift.
   D. By the order in which your co-worker does them.

5. Why is it critical to learn time management skills?
   A. So you never have to come in on your day off.
   B. So you have time to meet each resident's needs.
   C. So that you can leave work early when you want.
   D. So you have a chance to be employee of the month.

ACTIVITY 3 – PRIORITIZING CARE

Decide which resident you should care for first and place a 1 by their name, a 2 by the resident you would assist next, and a 3 by the name of the resident you would assist last.

Case Study A

It is 8 a.m. and three residents need your attention all at once:

1. _____ Mrs. Siegelman is going to the hospital for an MRI at 9:30 a.m. She needs assistance bathing and dressing.

2. _____ Mr. Riley is anxious to take part in an activity later this morning. He needs your assistance to change clothes and has already asked for your help twice.

3. _____ Mrs. Byrne is confined to bed and has mild dementia. She hasn't eaten her breakfast yet because she needs assistance with feeding.

Case Study B

It is 5:45 p.m. and the evening is not going smoothly:

1. _____ Mr. Sessions is going to dinner with his daughter at 6 p.m. He was ready to go when he had an accident in his pants.

2. _____ Mrs. Miller was admitted today. Dinner is already being served in the dining room, and she won't come out of her room.

3. _____ Mr. Dupree has just returned from a visit with his grandchildren and has vomited on himself and the hallway floor.

Case Study C

It is 6 a.m. and your shift is going to be busy up until the end:

1. _____ Mrs. Harrison began coughing up blood during the night. Her son will arrive shortly to take her to the hospital for tests. She needs assistance dressing.

2. _____ Mrs. Daugherty has been up all night and seems agitated. She is at the desk asking for coffee.

3. _____ Mr. Lucas has moderate dementia. He has taken all his paja-mas off and is standing in the doorway of the tub room.

ACTIVITY 4 – MATCHING

Read the descriptions of residents you've been assigned to care for on your shift. You need information from the charge nurse before you begin providing care. In the space provided, write the letter of the question that pertains to that resident.

Resident	Question for the Charge Nurse
1. _E_ You will care for Mrs. Dahlgren this evening. At report you learned she only ate 50% of her breakfast and didn't touch her lunch.	A. Is this resident able to ambulate with assistance?
2. _A_ You learned at report that Mr. Simmons was up all night. He has orders to go to physical therapy in the morning and you usually assist him with walking two times each day.	B. Should this resident receive the usual amount of exercise today?
3. _B_ Mrs. Mattson had hip replacement surgery. She has been going to physical therapy once a day and sitting up in a chair for two hours each day. You are supposed to assist her with walking, but yesterday she refused to walk.	C. Is it o.k. for this resident to eat?
4. _D_ Mrs. Jackson has complained of a stomach ache all day. She states that she is hungry now and would like to eat dinner.	D. Should I offer this resident a snack before dinner?
5. _C_ Mr. Rutledge is having surgery in the morning. He is NPO after midnight.	E. Is there anything I should do for this resident this evening?

ACTIVITY 5 – PRIORITIZING TASKS

For each situation below, decide the order in which tasks should be completed. Write a 1 beside the task you would do first, a 2 beside the task you would do next, and a 3 by the task you would do last. Any task you put off to the last may have to be done by the next shift.

Task List A

It is 6 a.m. and you must complete the following tasks:

1. _1_ Mrs. Neilsen is having minor surgery today. She will be picked up at 8 a.m. You have to assist her with bathing and dressing.

2. _3_ You must complete the 24-hour intake and output records for all your residents.

3. _2_ Three of your residents rise around 6 a.m. and like to receive a.m. care right away.

Task List B

It is 1 p.m. and you must complete the following tasks:

1. _1_ Give supplements to three residents and monitor their intake.

2. _2_ Assist two residents with walking.

3. _3_ Transfer vital signs and input/output information from your note pad to the appropriate charts.

Task List C

It is 10:30 p.m. and you must complete the following tasks:

1. ___ Offer a snack and beverage *bebida* to three residents who are NPO after midnight.

2. ___ Change the linens on an empty bed after a pitcher of water was accidentally spilled on them.

3. ___ Sit with a resident whose son just passed away suddenly.

ACTIVITY 6 – RESPONSIBILITY REVIEW

1. Give an example of a shift-related responsibility for the 7 a.m. to 3:30 p.m. shift.

2. Give an example of a shift-related responsibility for the 3 p.m. to 11:30 p.m. shift.

3. Give an example of a shift-related responsibility for the 11 p.m. to 7:30 a.m. shift.

ACTIVITY 7 – QUESTION & ANSWER

Using your own words, write an answer to each question.

1. What must you do before you can put a plan in place for providing care?

_____

_____

_____

_____

_____

2. What does it mean to prioritize?

_____

_____

_____

_____

_____

3. How well do you manage your time and yourself? Consider your personal and professional responsibilities, then develop a plan and write it below.

_____

_____

_____

_____

_____

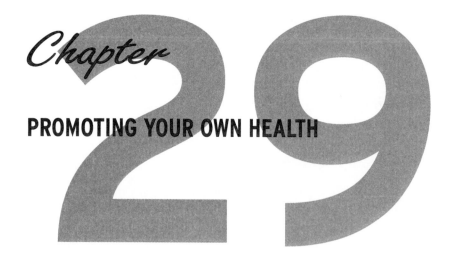

Chapter 29

PROMOTING YOUR OWN HEALTH

ACTIVITY 1 – MATCHING

In the space provided, write the letter of the correct definition.

Term	Definition
1. _E_ Aerobic	A. A mental state; the way life is viewed
2. _B_ Anaerobic	B. Exercise that does not increase the supply of oxygen to the body tissue
3. _A_ Attitude	C. A way of living
4. _D_ Health promotion	D. Process of working to achieve a state of health and well-being
5. _C_ Healthy lifestyle	E. Steady exercise that increases the heart rate and the amount of oxygen delivered to body tissue

ACTIVITY 2 – CONTENT REVIEW

List eight lifestyle factors that can influence your health. Refer to the textbook if necessary. Hint: one lifestyle factor is to wear your seatbelt.

1. _____

2. _____

3. _____

4. _____

5. _____

6. _____

7. _____

8. _____

List five ways to keep a positive attitude. Refer to the textbook if necessary. Hint: one way is to "see the glass half full, not half empty."

9. _____

10. _____

11. _____

12. _____

13. _____

ACTIVITY 3 – MULTIPLE CHOICE

Circle the letter beside the best answer.

1. Complete the following sentence. Good health depends on:
   A. Eating liver and spinach everyday.
   B. Drinking 8 oz of orange juice everyday.
   C. Staying very thin and avoiding carbohydrates.
   D. Good nutrition, regular exercise, and a positive attitude.

2. According to the food pyramid, which food group is considered a grain?
   A. Pasta
   B. Peas
   C. Oranges
   D. Beans

3. Women should limit their alcohol consumption to no more than:
   A. 1 drink per day
   B. 2 drinks per day
   C. 1 drink per week
   D. 2 drinks per week

4. What does the word "aerobic" mean?
   A. Healthy.
   B. With oxygen.
   C. Without oxygen.
   D. Outdoor activity.

5. When you exercise regularly, you help maintain joint flexibility and mobility. What kinds of problems can flexibility and mobility prevent?
   A. Poor vision.
   B. Skin cancer.
   C. Contractures.
   D. Forgetfulness.
   (esquecimento)

ACTIVITY 4 – CONTENT REVIEW

In the left hand column, list the five food groups from the USDA food pyramid. In the right hand column, list the amount you should eat daily of that category. Use your textbook if necessary.

Food Group   Servings

1a. _____   1b. _____

2a. _____   2b. _____

3a. _____   3b. _____

4a. _____   4b. _____

5a. _____   5b. _____

ACTIVITY 5 – HABITS TO CONSIDER

For two days, keep a journal and write down everything that you eat, the exercise you get, and special activities that you enjoy. After two days, make lists of the following:

1. What I can do to exercise:

   _____

   _____

   _____

2. How I can improve what I eat:

   _____

   _____

   _____

3. Nice things I can do for myself:

   _____

   _____

   _____

ACTIVITY 6 – CRITICAL THINKING

List some reasons why you think some people do not live a healthy lifestyle. For each of the reasons you list, describe a way to change. Note the example provided.

No time to exercise.   *Take a walk at lunchtime instead of eating dessert.*

_____

_____

_____

_____

_____

In your own words, describe good nutrition.

_____

_____

_____

_____

Describe the benefits of exercise.

_____

_____

_____

_____

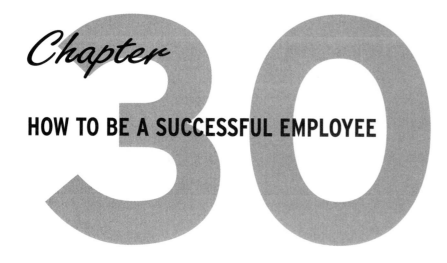

HOW TO BE A SUCCESSFUL EMPLOYEE

ACTIVITY 1 – SPELL IT OUT

Using the terms and clues provided complete the spelling of each word.

4 Aggressive   2 Assertive   1 Competency   3 Initiative

1. Abilities that are legally required or shown to be adequate: ___ ___ M ___ ___ ___ ___ ___ N ___ ___ ___

2. Behavior in which you speak up for yourself without hurting others: ___ ___ S ___ ___ ___ ___ ___ E

3. Attempting to take the first step to settle an issue: ___ ___ ___ I ___ ___ ___ ___ ___ ___ V ___

4. Behavior that is hurtful to others and may make them angry: ___ ___ ___ ___ R ___ ___ S ___ ___ ___ ___

ACTIVITY 2 – TRUE/FALSE

Read each statement. In the space provided, write T if the statement is true or F if the statement is false.

1. T   Once a nurse assistant has passed the state exam, they know everything they need to do their job.

2. T   Most nurse assistants who do well in training also do well on the state exam. ?

3. T   No matter who you are or how much you know, you always can learn something new.

4. F   For most people, starting a new job isn't stressful.

5. F   For a nurse assistant, the chain of command begins with the director of food services.

6. T   When you act assertively, you always get what you want.

7. F   When you act aggressively, people will respect you.

8. T   Feedback from residents and co-workers can help you improve your work.

ACTIVITY 3 – CONTENT REVIEW

Complete each list, referring to your textbook as needed.

Part A

List five steps you can take to keep yourself motivated on the job. Hint: one step is to stay healthy.

1. _____

2. _____

3. _____

4. _____

5. _____

Part B

List five habits that can make your job unpleasant. Hint: one habit is gossiping about residents or staff.

1. _____

2. _____

3. _____

4. _____

5. _____

ACTIVITY 4 – YES OR NO

Read over the following suggestions for preparing for the state exam. If it is an effective strategy, write YES in the space provided. If it is a not an effective strategy, write NO.

1. Y Get a good night's sleep before the exam.

2. Y Have all the necessary documents with you.

3. Y Eat a well-balanced meal before the exam.

4. Y Practice skills with a friend or co-worker.

5. N Have several glasses of wine to relax you before the exam.

6. N Obtain a sample test and complete it.

7. Y Review the text and what you learned during training.

8. N Cross your fingers and hope for the best.

ACTIVITY 5 – MULTIPLE CHOICE

Circle the letter beside the best answer.

1. How can you create a good first impression with a potential employer?
   A. Take a box of candy as a gesture of friendship.
   B. Take your best friend with you when you interview.
   C. Fill out the employment application neatly and accurately.
   D. Tell them what you didn't like about your previous supervisors.

2. Once you begin working as a nurse assistant, you can expect to:
   A. Know everything you need to know.
   B. Receive an orientation to the new job.
   C. Feel completely comfortable in your new role.
   D. Feel completely at ease with residents and families the first day.

3. How can you stay motivated on the job?
   A. Do no more than what the job requires.
   B. Take advantage of all opportunities to learn.
   C. Ignore the people and co-workers you don't like.
   D. Find a resident who will listen to your complaints.

4. Following the chain of command, what is your first step in resolving a grievance or concern about your work?
   A. Talking to the housekeeper.
   B. Talking to the charge nurse.
   C. Talking to the social worker.
   D. Talking to the administrator.

5. What is the best way to know if you're doing a good job?
   A. Assume that people will tell you if you make a mistake.
   B. Do your job the way other nurse assistants do theirs.
   C. Ask residents, families, and co-workers for feedback.
   D. Ask others to complete a survey about your performance.

ACTIVITY 6 –MATCHING

Read each statement or action. In the space provided, write AG if the statement or action is aggressive, AS if it is assertive, or P if it is passive.

AGGRESSIVE   ASSERTIVE   PASSIVE

You work the evening shift and you've completed all the normal tasks before taking your dinner break. You've helped all of your residents get ready for bed, passed around snacks and supplements, and completed your paperwork. Your co-worker is running behind schedule. You've seen her chatting on the phone and watched her flip through a magazine in the break room. Now she has asked if you will help her complete her tasks so the two of you can go to dinner together. You are hungry and you resent the fact that she's wasted her time while you made good use of yours.

1. AS *suspira encolhe os ombros* You sigh and shrug your shoulders, put your dinner away, and ask her what needs to be done.

2. P You explain that you've completed your work and that you're going to take your break now.

3. AG You shake your finger in her face as you tell her that you've watched her waste time all evening and that it's not your responsibility to help her do her job.

Mrs. Lane's daughter discovers that one of her mother's nicest dresses has a rip in it. Mrs. Lane, who is confused, tells the daughter you caused the tear. You have no idea how or when the dress was torn.

4. _____ You say, "I have no idea when or how it was torn, but I'm sorry it happened to such a pretty dress. Would you like to talk to the charge nurse about this?"

5. _____ You say, "Your mother doesn't have a clue what's going on around her, so how can you accuse me of tearing the dress? If you don't like the way I do my job, you should speak to the charge nurse."

6. _____ You say, "It was probably my fault. I'm really sorry."

ACTIVITY 7 – QUESTIONS TO CONSIDER

Using your own words, answer the following questions.

As a result of taking this course, what new information did you learn about residents in nursing facilities?

_____

_____

_____

What new information did you learn about yourself?

_____

_____

_____

What can you do if you find yourself unhappy in your job?

_____

_____

_____

What are some ways you can continue to learn on the job?

_____

_____

_____

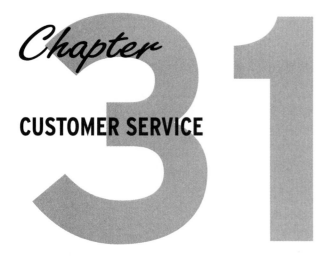

Chapter 31

CUSTOMER SERVICE

ACTIVITY 1 – WORD SCRAMBLE

Unscramble each word in the following phrases to spell key concepts discussed in this chapter.

Nonverbal Communication 3
Customer Service 1
Verbal Communication 2

1. rceumsot veciesr

   ___ ___ ___ ___ ___ ___ ___   ___ ___ ___ ___ ___ ___ ___

2. blavre mictanocmuaino

   ___ ___ ___ ___ ___ ___

   ___ ___ ___ ___ ___ ___ ___ ___ ___ ___ ___ ___ ___

3. vnolernba ncomomituanic

   ___

ACTIVITY 2 – DO-DON'T SITUATIONS

Write either "Do" or "Don't" before each of the following statements as appropriate.

1. ____ listen attentively to all concerns.

2. ____ talk about co-workers in private so that you will not hurt their feelings.

3. ____ share all the information that you know about residents so that all will be Informed.

4. ____ honor your commitments to complaining families.

5. ____ use common slang so that everyone will understand what you are talking about.

6. ____ provide individualized care to residents only if they are able to communicate their wishes.

7. ____ take differences personally.

8. ____ be open to the ideas of others.

9. ____ offer resident choices only when they are not demented.

10. ____ provide consistent care but be flexible with the wishes of the resident.

ACTIVITY 3 – MATCHING

In the space provided, write the letter of the behavior that matches the concept.

1. ____ Remember your manners

2. ____ People come first

3. ____ Don't use technical language

4. ____ Don't rush

5. ____ Don't be too busy to be nice

6. ____ Be friendly always

A. Take time to get information

B. "There ya go" is not "Thank you"

C. Don't give short answers

D. Explain unfamiliar words

E. Residents' behavior reflects how they are treated

F. Give the resident your complete attention

ACTIVITY 4 – CRITICAL CUSTOMER SITUATIONS

1. Describe five ways that you can incorporate customer service and mindful caregiving into ADL care for the resident.

2. Discuss at least three different socialization techniques that you can use during mealtime and dining.

3. Give at least three examples of things that you can do to include customer service and specialized care into resident activities.

4. Describe a situation when you have had to deal with someone who was unhappy with a service or product and describe how you handled it. How did you feel? What could you have done differently that would have made the situation better?

Adaptability
AHCA
Balance
CNA
Empathy
Enthusiasm
Nonverbal
Ownership
Resiliency
Responsibility

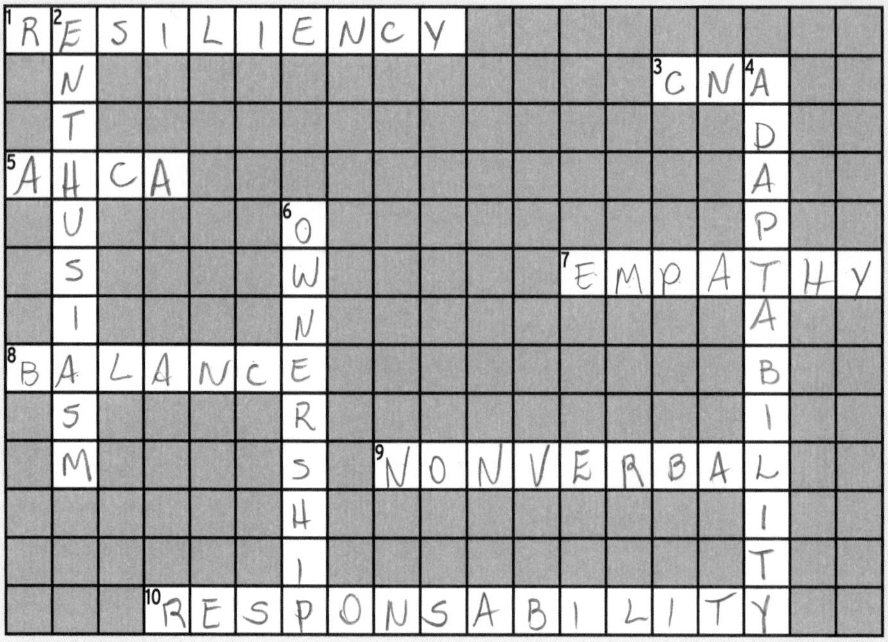

Crossword grid (handwritten answers):
- 1 across: RESILIENCY
- 2 down: ENTHUSIASM
- 3 across: CNA
- 4 down: ADAPTABILITY
- 5 across: AHCA
- 6 down: OWNERSHIP
- 7 across: EMPATHY
- 8 across: BALANCE
- 9 across: NONVERBAL
- 10 across: RESPONSABILITY

ACROSS

1. Characteristic of being able to bounce back from adversity _saltar pl tras_

3. Certified Nursing Assistant

5. American Health Care Association

7. The ability to understand, be aware of, and be sensitive to the feelings, thoughts, and experiences of others _ciente_

8. Satisfying the customer while keeping the organization's best interest

9. Communication by rolling the eyes

10. Characteristic of living up to the duties that one accepts _deveres_

DOWN

2. Characteristic of having a strong interest and bringing energy to a project or service

4. Characteristic of being flexible to effectively deal with different customers and situations

6. Being committed to solving a problem or taking it to someone who will

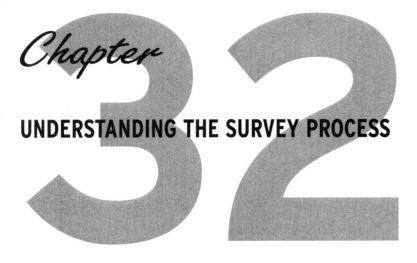

Chapter 32

UNDERSTANDING THE SURVEY PROCESS

ACTIVITY 1 – WORD SEARCH

Find and circle the following words in the word search grid below. (Words may be sideways, up and down, or diagonal, and may be spelled backwards.)

ANNUAL	FOLLOW-UP	QIS
COMPLAINT	INITIAL	QUALITY
EMOTIONS	INTERVIEW	RESIDENT
EXIT	LIFE	SAFETY
FAMILY	OBSERVE	TRADITIONAL

```
O   S   C   Y   X   Y   S   W   I   C   S   A   V   D   R

O   B   N   P   X   A   Y   N   O   O   I   V   Q   R   A

P   R   S   O   F   T   T   F   Q   M   Q   Z   A   X   N

U   D   X   E   I   E   L   R   D   P   L   J   Y   X   N

N   E   T   L   R   T   Z   L   B   L   A   D   K   R   U

G   Y   A   V   F   V   O   H   A   A   I   Y   M   S   A

R   U   I   K   X   A   E   M   I   I   T   S   A   G   L

Q   E   A   K   S   G   M   T   E   N   I   E   V   Z   W

W   R   O   L   G   O   W   I   P   T   N   E   D   Z   T

B   E   C   E   X   P   D   B   L   O   I   N   F   I   T

I   R   E   G   U   O   B   B   C   Y   N   P   B   I   C

F   O   L   L   O   W   U   P   N   F   Q   V   E   G   L

T   C   W   U   L   K   C   Z   M   N   H   A   T   X   Z

T   N   E   D   I   S   E   R   T   I   X   E   Y   J   E

Y   X   D   T   R   A   D   I   T   I   O   N   A   L   C
```

ACTIVITY 2 – QIS OR TRADITIONAL SURVEY?

Write a Q of T before each of the following descriptions.

1. _____ Large sample of staff and residents
2. _____ Observation focused
3. _____ Interview focused
4. _____ More deficiencies expected
5. _____ Small sample size of staff and residents
6. _____ Surveyors in facility longer
7. _____ Surveyors for a shorter time in facility
8. _____ Fewer deficiencies expected
9. _____ Must have special training to implement
10. _____ Newest survey method

ACTIVITY 3 – FILL IN THE BLANK

Complete each sentence by adding the correct term.

Exit conference 5
Initial 3
Life Safety 1
Quality indicator survey 4
Quality measures 2

1. Rules for safety in a facility are called

   _____ _____ .

2. Surveyors review the facility's history and _____ _____ documents before coming to the facility.

3. During the _____ stage, surveyors explain their reason for being there and any complaints that they will be reviewing.

4. QIS stands for _____ _____

   _____ .

5. The final conference with the administrator and the surveyors is called the _____ _____ .

ACTIVITY 4 – MULTIPLE CHOICE

Circle the letter by the best answer.

1. The initial tour is designed to:
   A. Make an initial review of the facility, residents, and environment
   B. Make a determination to grant the facility another license to admit residents
   C. To go over quality data with rest of the staff
   D. Deliver the plan of correction to the charge nurses

2. Which is an example of emotional or behavioral reactions?
   A. Edema
   B. Poor oral care
   C. Resident yelling
   D. Weight loss

3. Which is an example of an environmental/safety concern for surveyors?
   A. Handwashing
   B. Pulling the curtain for privacy
   C. Availability of scheduled activities
   D. Resident choices for bath times

4. Which is an example of a question that could be asked of staff?
   A. Do you have privacy when speaking on the phone?
   B. Is the food served the way that you like it?
   C. What would you do if you witnessed abuse?
   D. Do you get to choose what you want to wear?

5. What is an example of a question that could be asked of a resident or family member?
   A. What would you do in case of a fire?
   B. How do you know if someone is on isolation precautions?
   C. How do people act toward you when they are giving you care?
   D. How do you know the facility policies?

Write the answers in the space provided. Refer to the textbook if necessary.

1. Name four sources of information that are reviewed during a survey.
    a. _____
    b. _____
    c. _____
    d. _____

2. Name three different reasons for a survey and explain each.
    a. _____
    b. _____
    c. _____

3. Give examples of four quality of life issues that surveyors will be observing.
    a. _____
    b. _____
    c. _____
    d. _____

4. Give examples of at least five care areas that surveyors will consider upon their visit.
    a. _____
    b. _____
    c. _____
    d. _____
    e. _____

5. What are examples of three things that you can do during a survey to fulfill your role?
    a. _____
    b. _____
    c. _____

Practice Exam

Circle the letter beside the best answer.

1. Which of these services is usually provided in a long term care facility?
   - A. Home health care.
   - B. Radiation therapy.
   - C. Rehabilitative care.
   - D. Surgery.

2. What is an example of mindful caregiving?
   - A. Being on time for work.
   - B. Encouraging residents to wear clothing you like.
   - C. Observing changes in a resident's mood or routine.
   - D. Requiring a resident to stick with the facility's schedule.

3. What is an effective way to get to know a resident?
   - A. Discuss the resident with housekeeping staff.
   - B. Read the resident's mail and personal papers.
   - C. Ask the resident about their needs and preferences.
   - D. Check with the resident's roommate for information.

4. Which of these is an example of negligence?
   - A. Teasing a resident in an unkind manner.
   - B. Threatening a resident with physical harm.
   - C. Locking a resident in their room against their will.
   - D. Not taking a resident to the bathroom when they ask.

5. Which of these statements about our perceptions is true?
   - A. Our perceptions about residents are always accurate.
   - B. We should always believe that what we perceive is true, regardless of whether it may be right or wrong.
   - C. Our perceptions influence how we behave toward others.
   - D. Single-minded perceptions of residents help us get to know them better.

6. How can you make a new resident feel that they belong?
   - A. Call them by the nickname "honey."
   - B. Encourage them to participate in activities.
   - C. Ask if you can borrow some of their jewelry.
   - D. Leave them alone to adjust to the facility on their own.

7. Which of the following symptoms is typical of mid-stage dementia?
   - A. Loss of appetite.
   - B. Tendency to feel cold most of the time.
   - C. Great difficulty making decisions.
   - D. Improved recent memory.

8. Which of these nonverbal behaviors helps develop a positive relationship with a resident?
   - A. Smiling warmly.
   - B. Always keeping your facial expressions neutral.
   - C. Looking over the resident's shoulder when you speak to them.
   - D. Folding your arms across your chest.

9. What is the purpose of a living will?
   - A. To settle property and financial issues when a person dies.
   - B. To help family members decide how they want their loved one cared for.
   - C. To keep family members away from a dying resident.
   - D. To guide decisions about a person's care if they become incapacitated.

10. You're involved in an argument with a co-worker. In order to resolve the conflict, you should:
    - A. Tell the co-worker what's wrong with their point of view.
    - B. Bring up past conflicts you've had with the co-worker.
    - C. Take time to understand the other person's point of view.
    - D. Calm things down by joking about their point of view.

11. A resident's care plan is used as a tool to:
    - A. Determine whether the resident qualifies for Medicaid payments.
    - B. Invite family members to facility parties.
    - C. Plan for new building improvements.
    - D. Coordinate all treatments and services for the resident.

12. How residents perceive and respond to pain is influenced by:
    - A. Their nutritional status.
    - B. Sunlight.
    - C. The clothing they are wearing at the time.
    - D. Their cultural or religious background and beliefs.

13. Whenever you prepare to do a task, you should ask yourself a number of questions, including which of the following?
    - A. Is this task in my job description?
    - B. Did I get the resident's permission to do the task?
    - C. Should I call the resident's family to check whether they want me to do this task?
    - D. Will the charge nurse respect me more for doing this task?

14. You can help to break the chain of infection at each link by:
    - A. Sterilizing all bed linen every morning.
    - B. Disinfecting all surfaces.
    - C. Wearing a gown and protective eyewear at all times.
    - D. Washing your hands before and after every contact with a resident.

15. When a family member is angry or critical, you should:
    A. Take their comments personally.
    B. Explain that the facility is understaffed and there's nothing anyone can do.
    X C. Be supportive and report the situation to the charge nurse.
    D. Pretend you agree with them that the facility is not doing a good job.

16. Your role in helping maintain a resident's nutrition includes:
    A. Planning meals for the week.
    B. Helping food service staff prepare meals.
    C. Insisting that residents eat everything on their plate.
    X D. Serving meals while hot foods are still hot and cold foods are cold.

17. To make sure a resident is safe during a bath, you should:
    A. Close the tub room door.
    B. Undress the resident in the tub room.
    X C. Check the water temperature.
    D. Remove all your jewelry.

18. As a nurse assistant, you typically learn about a resident's symptoms by:
    A. Interviewing the resident's roommate.
    X B. Talking to the resident.
    C. Observing the resident while they sleep.
    D. Taking the resident's vital signs.

19. Which of the following occurs because of nervous system changes as we age?
    A. Slowing of respirations.
    B. Slowing of heartbeat.
    C. Decreased insulin production.
    X D. Decreased short-term memory.

20. The Heimlich maneuver is used with a resident who is:
    A. Vomiting.
    B. Having a seizure.
    C. Choking.
    D. Feeling nauseous.

21. How can you help a resident be independent?
    A. Select their clothing for them each day.
    X B. Encourage the resident to do what they can.
    C. Insist on helping them with bathing.
    D. Leave them alone to take care of themselves.

22. The Resident's Bill of Rights includes:
    A. The right to have a private room.
    B. The right to be happy all the time.
    X C. The right to privacy and confidentiality.
    D. The right to receive all services free of charge.

23. The nurse asks you to give ROM exercise to a resident who is confined to bed. According to her care plan, there are no restrictions. What does "no restrictions" mean?
    A. You should work their joints and muscles very hard.
    B. Provide ROM exercise as often as possible on each shift.
    ? C. The resident should be able to do all of the exercises alone.
    X D. You may move each joint through its full available range.

24. Mr. Nathanson is experiencing a seizure and you have called for help. What else should you do for him?
    A. Pour water into his mouth.
    X B. Help him to the floor to prevent a fall.
    C. Put a toothbrush or something firm between his teeth for him to bite on.
    D. Ask other residents to help you hold him down firmly.

25. When you maintain the resident's privacy during all aspects of personal care, which theme of care are you paying attention to?
    X A. Respect.
    B. Safety.
    C. Communication.
    D. Infection control.

26. Using good body mechanics will help you:
    A. Get all your work done before your shift ends.
    B. Lose weight.
    X C. Avoid injuries.
    D. Develop stronger muscles.

27. You should check a resident's vital signs:
    A. Only on the first day of each month.
    X B. Whenever a change occurs that might signal an illness.
    C. Everyday at the beginning of your shift.
    D. Whenever you feel like it.

28. If a resident starts to feel dizzy as you help them stand up from their bed to get to their walker, you should:
    A. Move them quickly to the walker before they have a chance to fall.
    X B. Help them to lie down in bed and call for the charge nurse.
    C. Keep them standing for a minute until the dizziness passes.
    D. Have them sit on the edge of the bed while you go to talk to the charge nurse.

29. Your role in the care plan meeting includes:
    A. Sharing information about the resident.
    B. Serving coffee and doughnuts to the interdisciplinary team.
    C. Deciding which doctors and nurses should attend.
    D. Diagnosing the resident's medical condition.

30. When you position a resident on their side, their legs should normally be positioned:
    A. With a pillow between them.
    B. However you think.
    C. With both legs straight and slightly apart.
    D. With one leg straight and one leg slightly bent.

31. When you provide personal care, it is important to:
    A. Have all morning care done before 8 a.m.
    B. Never give care that has not been clearly requested by the family.
    C. Keep on schedule, even if you have to rush slow residents.
    D. Encourage the resident to do all that they can for themselves.

32. How can you help a family get over their guilt when a resident is admitted into a long-term care facility?
    A. Encourage them to question their decision to admit their family member.
    B. Give their family member the best care you can.
    C. Tell them they are in charge of bathing and dressing their family member whenever they visit.
    D. Just nod and smile whenever they make suggestions about their loved one's care.

33. What is a common cause of a decubitus ulcer?
    A. Uncomfortable clothing.
    B. Dirty pajamas.
    C. Pressure on the skin.
    D. Stress caused by family arguments.

34. What is a benefit of observing residents carefully while providing personal care?
    A. It frees you from having to observe residents at other times.
    B. You have the opportunity to talk with residents about family members.
    C. You may note both physical and psychological changes in residents.
    D. You can decide whether or not to give residents their medications, depending on how they feel.

35. Why is it important reason to make a neat, wrinkle free bed?
    A. Wrinkles give germs places to grow.
    B. It is more difficult to launder sheets that become very wrinkled.
    C. Wrinkled sheets can cause skin irritation and breakdown.
    D. Old-fashioned charge nurses think neat beds look better.

36. The signs and symptoms of dehydration may include:
    A. Blurred vision.
    B. Rosy pink skin color.
    C. Decreased urine output.
    D. Elevated blood pressure.

37. Why is it important to be familiar with a resident's elimination pattern?
    A. So that you never have to clean up an accident.
    B. So that you can recognize and report any changes.
    C. To keep the family informed at every visit.
    D. Because you discuss every resident's elimination at the end of your shift.

38. Why is it good practice to use a guard belt when transferring a resident?
    A. You never need other helpers.
    B. It helps to support the resident's body during the transfer.
    C. It keeps the resident's clothing in place during the transfer.
    D. It makes the transfer go twice as fast.

39. You are a new nurse assistant at your facility. How might you learn that a certain resident has frequent incontinence?
    A. By checking the resident's medical record.
    B. By interviewing all family members that come to visit the resident.
    C. By sneaking into the resident's room at lunch to check the sheets for dampness.
    D. By asking the laundry to check the resident's clothing for urine stains.

40. When you give ROM exercises, it is important to:
    A. Wear gloves and a gown.
    B. Exercise the resident at least until they begin to sweat.
    C. Follow the therapist's written plan.
    D. Move each joint just to the point where it begins to be painful.

41. What is an ICF/MR?
    A. A nursing facility that cares for residents who are mentally retarded.
    B. A specialized facility that provides care for an elderly disabled person.
    C. A congregate care facility for elderly residents with diabetes.
    D. A facility that provides a home-like environment for people in wheelchairs.

42. A resident's daughter complains to you that you ask her mother to bathe herself. How should you answer the daughter?
    A. You have a lot of people to care for and don't have time for everyone.
    B. You suggest the daughter care for the mother herself.
    C. You ask the daughter file a formal complaint.
    D. You explain you are helping her mother maintain her independence.

43. You are communicating assertively when you:
    A. Feel guilty after saying you cannot volunteer for an extra shift.
    B. Share your complaints with residents.
    C. Speak up for yourself without hurting others.
    D. Say what you think other people will want to hear.

44. To prevent a stage one pressure ulcer from getting worse, you should:
    A. Frequently give the resident ice chips to suck on.
    B. Give the resident three vitamin pills daily.
    C. Follow the charge nurse's instructions.
    D. Cover the area with a warm, moist cloth at all times.

45. When a resident with an infection is on contact precautions, you should:
    A. Never allow any visitors under any circumstances.
    B. Request that the charge nurse provide all care.
    C. Wear gloves when providing care.
    D. Install a special air ventilation system.

46. Which of the following techniques is helpful when you are dealing with an agitated resident?
    A. Yelling.
    B. Distraction.
    C. Reality orientation.
    D. Clapping your hands and stomping your foot.

47. Which of the following is a developmentally disabled person?
    A. A person who lost use of their legs after a car accident.
    B. An elderly person who has developed Alzheimer's disease.
    C. A person with a chronic, severe condition that developed in childhood.
    D. A frail elderly person who needs assistance with bathing and dressing.

48. You can help a dying resident cope with their feelings by:
    A. Discouraging them from talking about painful topics.
    B. Using techniques of reality orientation.
    C. Explaining your own views about death.
    D. Listening to what they have to say.

49. After you make rounds, you prioritize your tasks based on:
    A. Which tasks require the most supplies.
    B. Which tasks can be completed most quickly.
    C. What tasks you'll have to leave for the next shift.
    D. Which residents require the most assistance.

50. How can you demonstrate your desire to be a good employee?
    A. Be late to work no more than once a week.
    B. Record care activities in the resident's medical record even before you have done them.
    C. Cooperate with other team members.
    D. Offer to share your lunch with other nurse assistants.

51. You should limit your daily intake of carbohydrates to one serving of meat, poultry, fish, dry beans, or nuts. One serving means
    A. 2-3 once of cooked lean meat.
    B. 1 lb of cooked dry beans.
    C. four eggs.
    D. 3 tablespoons of peanut butter.

52. What is "mindful caregiving"?
    A. Wearing comfortable shoes and clothing to work.
    B. Storing soiled equipment and supplies in the clean supply room.
    C. Paying attention to details and being open, observant, and flexible.
    D. Sharing your opinions about a resident's care with their family members.

53. Aging changes happen to everyone. Which of these changes is also
a normal part of aging?
A. The need to be fed.
B. An inability to walk.
X. Thinning of the skin.
D. The loss of one's teeth.

54. Walkers, canes, and crutches are examples of which type of device?
A. Orthotic.
X. Assistive.
C. Listening.
D. Prosthetic.

55. When caring for a resident you must consider:
A. Your own schedule.
B. Your own preferences.
X. The resident's preferences.
D. The housekeeping schedule.

56. a history of a resident includes both _____ and
_____ information.

57. A physical exam proceeds through each _____
_____.

58. A program with a specially trained interdisciplinary team that cares
for a terminally ill resident who is expected to die within 6 months
is called haspice .

59. Blood sugar is lowered by the person receiving _____
_____.

60. Oxygen assists the person with emphysema pulmonar
_____ · lung diasese

Answer Sheet

1. _____	31. _____
2. _____	32. _____
3. _____	33. _____
4. _____	34. _____
5. _____	35. _____
6. _____	36. _____
7. _____	37. _____
8. _____	38. _____
9. _____	39. _____
10. _____	40. _____
11. _____	41. _____
12. _____	42. _____
13. _____	43. _____
14. _____	44. _____
15. _____	45. _____
16. _____	46. _____
17. _____	47. _____
18. _____	48. _____
19. _____	49. _____
20. _____	50. _____
21. _____	51. _____
22. _____	52. _____
23. _____	53. _____
24. _____	54. _____
25. _____	55. _____
26. _____	56. _____
27. _____	57. _____
28. _____	58. _____
29. _____	59. _____
30. _____	60. _____

Appendix

SKILLS CHECKLISTS

HANDWASHING (CHAPTER 9)

Note: *Check the sink, soap dispenser, and towel dispenser before beginning. Ask yourself: "Will I contaminate my hands touching these items after I wash my hands?" If your answer is yes, prepare these before you begin.*

1. _____ Remove your watch and roll up your sleeves. **Note:** *You may not want to wear jewelry so you don't have to constantly remove it for handwashing. If you do not remove your watch and rings, be sure to wash, rinse, and dry under them.*
2. _____ Turn on the water to a comfortable temperature. Wet your hands and wrists.
3. _____ Apply soap to your hands.
4. _____ Rub your hands together in a circular motion with friction for at least 20 seconds. Lace your fingers together to wash in between them).
   Clean under your fingernails: Use a nail brush or orange stick, or rub your nails briskly in your palm to clean them. **Note:** *Because acrylic or silk-wrap (artificial) nails are difficult to clean under and may harbor bacteria, they should not be worn.*
5. _____ Rinse your hands with warm water, keeping them downward, allowing the water to run from the wrist to the fingers.
6. _____ Get paper towels from the dispenser. **Note:** *If you have to touch the dispenser to remove the towel, you must have the towel ready before you start so you do not contaminate your hands.*
7. _____ Dry your hands with paper towels. Start at the top of the fingers and work downward toward the wrists.
8. _____ Turn off the faucets with a paper towel.
9. _____ Discard paper towels in appropriate receptacle.
10. _____ You should use a moisturizing lotion on your hands if they are dry.

PROCEDURE 11-1 – COLLECTING A SPUTUM SPECIMEN

Note: *Make sure a resident who chews tobacco has not done so before you collect the specimen. If the resident has just eaten, ask them to rinse out their mouth. Try to collect the specimen in the morning. Often large amounts of sputum are coughed up first thing in the morning.*

1. _____ Give the resident the sputum collection container or hold it yourself. Take care not to touch its inside surface, or lining.
2. _____ Ask the resident to take deep breaths and cough deeply from the chest. They may need to cough several times to get enough sputum for the sample. Ask them to try not to spit only saliva into the container.
3. _____ Place the lid securely on the specimen bottle. Label it with the resident's name, room number, and the date and time of the collection. Place the specimen in a biohazardous bag.
4. _____ Report the color, amount, and consistency of the specimen to the charge nurse.

PROCEDURE 11-2 – APPLICATION OF SUPPORT HOSE AND ELASTIC STOCKINGS

1. _____ Assist the person to lie on their backs.
2. _____ Expose only the person's legs.
3. _____ Clean and dry the person's legs and feet before applying elastic stockings.
4. _____ Apply a very small amount of baby powder to the person's legs and feet unless the person has any respiratory difficulty.
5. _____ Apply one elastic stocking at a time. Begin by rolling the stocking with your hands so that only the toe section is exposed. Put the stocking on the person's leg, positioning the hole over the top of the toes. Make sure the heel is properly placed. Then roll the stocking up the leg as far as it will go.
6. _____ Do the same on the other leg. The stockings should fit firmly and have no wrinkles.
7. _____ Check for good circulation and movement by observing the person's toes for color and ability to move freely.

PROCEDURE 11-3 – GIVING AN ENEMA

1. ____ Put on gloves.
2. ____ Place disposable protective pad under the resident's buttocks. Place a second protective pad at the end of the bed to place under and over bedpan when resident is finished.
3. ____ Position the resident on their left side, helping them turn if necessary. Make sure their hips are near the edge of the bed on the side where you're working.
4. ____ Hold the rectal tube over the bedpan. Open the clamp on the tubing and let the solution run through into the bedpan until it flows smoothly, so that no air is left in the tubing to cause discomfort for the resident. Close the clamp.
5. ____ Turn back the bath blanket so that the resident's hips are exposed but the rest of the body is covered. Hold the lubricated rectal tube about 5 inches from the tip. Gently put it into the rectum to the red line on the tube.
6. ____ Raise the container about 15 inches above the resident's hips. Never hold the container any higher.
7. ____ Open the clamp and let the solution run in slowly. If the resident complains of cramps, tell them to breathe deeply through their mouth, as you clamp the tubing for a minute or so. You may also lower the irrigating bag.
8. ____ When all the solution has run in, close the clamp.
9. ____ Remove the rectal tube. Place the tubing in a plastic trash bag.
10. ____ Turn the resident on their back and slip the bedpan under them. Ask the resident to try to hold the solution as long as possible. Raise the head of the bed. Ensure that the call button and toilet paper are within reach.
11. ____ Give the resident privacy, but do not leave them for a long period of time. Check on the resident after 5 minutes.
12. ____ When the resident feels they are done, put on gloves, and assist with wiping if necessary. Remove the bedpan and place it on a protective pad. Remove your gloves, and help the resident into a comfortable position. Put on gloves and remove the covered bedpan.

PROCEDURE 11-4 – APPLYING A DISPOSABLE INCONTINENCE BRIEF

1. ____ Place an incontinence pad on the bed to protect clean linen.
2. ____ Help the resident onto their back.
3. ____ Put on gloves.
4. ____ Help remove garments below the waist.
5. ____ Discard the soiled incontinence brief in the plastic trash bag.
6. ____ Remove and dispose of your soiled gloves.
7. ____ Put on new gloves.
8. ____ With the resident on their side, give perineal care, including cleaning the rectal area.
9. ____ Remove and dispose of your soiled gloves.
10. ____ Put on new gloves.
11. ____ Fan-fold one-half of the briefs under the resident's buttocks.
12. ____ Help the resident move onto their back. Unfold the side that was fan-folded, and open the adhesive tabs on both sides. Place the brief upward between the resident's legs, and join the tab from the back of the brief to the tab in the front of the brief.
13. ____ Put on the resident's underpants and clothing.

PROCEDURE 11-5 – EMPTYING A CATHETER DRAINAGE BAG

1. ____ Put on gloves.
2. ____ Place the paper towel on the floor underneath the drainage bag.
3. ____ Place the measuring container on the paper towel.
4. ____ The drainage bag has a closed clamp that allows the urine to flow from the bag. Open the clamp and drain all the urine into the container, making sure not to touch the clamp to the sides of the container.
5. ____ Close the clamp and secure it to the drainage bag immediately after it is completely drained.
6. ____ Note the amount of urine and discard the urine in the resident's toilet.
7. ____ Remove and discard your gloves, and wash your hands.
8. ____ Record the amount of urine on the intake and output record.

PROCEDURE 13-1 – TAKING AN ORAL TEMPERATURE

Note: *Check with the person to make sure they have not just eaten or drunk something hot or cold or smoked a cigarette in the last 10 minutes. These activities change the temperature of the mouth and give you a false reading. If they did, wait 5-10 minutes.*

1. _____ Shake the thermometer down to 95 F or to the lowest number, and then put on the plastic cover.
2. _____ Insert the bulb end of the thermometer under the resident's tongue, and ask them to close their lips around it. The resident may want to hold onto the end of the thermometer to keep it in place. The resident should not walk with the thermometer in their mouth.
3. _____ Wait at least 3 minutes. As you wait, you can take the person's pulse and respiratory rates. Remove the thermometer and the plastic cover. Read the temperature. **Note:** *If there is an excessive amount of mucus on the thermometer when you remove it, use a barrier such as gloves to remove the cover.*
4. _____ If you use an electronic thermometer, wait until it beeps.
5. _____ Record the result.

PROCEDURE 13-2 – TAKING A RECTAL TEMPERATURE

1. _____ Be sure to wear gloves.
2. _____ Shake down the thermometer to 95 F or lower.
3. _____ Position the resident on either side. Help the resident bend up the upper leg as far as possible.
4. _____ Put a plastic cover (if used) over the thermometer and lubricate it. Separate the person's buttocks with one hand while with the other you insert the bulb 1 inch into the rectum.
5. _____ Hold the thermometer in place 1 to 3 minutes, remove it, and wipe any excess lubricant from the rectum with a piece of tissue paper. Remove the cover, and read the thermometer.
6. _____ Record the result.

Note: *Always cover a resident while taking a rectal temperature. Never leave them during this time because they may roll off their side and be injured by the thermometer. Talk with the person while waiting for the temperature reading to take their mind off the procedure.*

PROCEDURE 13-3. – TAKING AN AXILLARY TEMPERATURE

1. _____ Shake down the thermometer to 95 F or lower.
2. _____ Loosen the resident's clothing to be able to reach the armpit. Dry the armpit.
3. _____ Place the thermometer in the resident's armpit. Have them place the arm down along their side.
4. _____ Wait 10 minutes. Remove the thermometer and read the temperature.
5. _____ Record the result.

PROCEDURE 13-4. – TAKING A RADIAL PULSE

1. _____ Place your second and third fingers gently over the radial artery (on the thumb side of the wrist) and note the rhythm of the pulse.
2. _____ Look at your watch, and when the second hand is on the 12, start counting the pulse for 1 minute. Count each beat you feel. Check for abnormalities in the rhythm.
3. _____ Record the result.

PROCEDURE 13-5. – TAKING A RESPIRATORY RATE

1. _____ Count the respiratory rate immediately after counting the pulse rate.
2. _____ Keep your fingers on the resident's radial pulse but without pressure. (Do this so the resident will breathe normally. Often residents hold their breath or breathe deeper if they know you are counting.) Watch the chest go up with inspiration and down with expiration.
3. _____ Count the respiratory rate for 1 minute.
4. _____ Record the result.

PROCEDURE 13-6. – TAKING A BLOOD PRESSURE

1. _____ Have the resident place their arm on the bed, bedside table, or arm of the chair, with their palm up and elbow at the same level as the heart. (If the arm is higher than the heart, the blood pressure can register too high. If the arm is lower than the heart, the blood pressure can register too low.)

2. _____ Expose the resident's arm by rolling the sleeve up to the shoulder, taking care that the sleeve is not too tight on the arm, which might increase the blood pressure. Wrap the blood pressure cuff evenly around the upper arm 1 inch above the elbow. Make sure the arm is not lying on the tubing and the tubing is not kinked. The tube that is attached to the bulb should be on the side closest to the resident's body. The tube to the sphygmomanometer gauge should be on the other side of the arm, away from the body. Be sure to use the correct size cuff for the resident. The wrong size cuff can give you an incorrect reading. The cuff should fit over the center of the resident's upper arm. It should not extend to the elbow or to under the resident's armpit.

3. _____ Close the valve in the air pump by turning it clockwise. The valve is the little metal knob on the bulb.

4. _____ Place the stethoscope earpieces in your ears.

5. _____ Locate the pulsation in the brachial artery by placing your second and third fingers over the area. When you find the pulse, place the diaphragm of the stethoscope firmly over the area and hold it in place with your left hand. Use your right hand if you are left-handed.

6. _____ With your right hand, pump air into the cuff by squeezing the bulb until the gauge measures 180–200.
   Note. *If you hear the pulse immediately after stopping pumping, begin again and pump the cuff so the gauge reads higher than 200 mm Hg (Hg=symbol for mercury). One way to avoid pumping the cuff too high is to feel the pulse at the brachial artery and pump the cuff slowly until you no longer feel the pulse, making sure to remember where you last felt the pulse and to add 30 mm Hg when beginning to take the blood pressure.*

7. _____ Slowly open the valve on the bulb and watch the cuff pressure decrease on the gauge.

8. _____ Listen for the first thumping sound and note the pressure reading; remember this number. This is the systolic pressure.

9. _____ Continue to listen for a distinct change in sound (muffled sounding) or the last sound and note the pressure reading. This is the diastolic pressure.

10. _____ Record the results.

PROCEDURE 13-7 – MEASURING HEIGHT AND WEIGHT USING AN UPRIGHT SCALE

1. _____ Determine if the resident can walk to the scale or whether you need to bring a portable scale to their room.

2. _____ Before they step on the scale, adjust the height measurement bar so it is higher than the resident's height.

3. _____ Ask the resident what their height is as a check for accuracy.

4. _____ Clear the scale and make sure it is balanced. It should register 0 when the weights are moved all the way over to the left.

5. _____ Place a paper towel on the scale platform. Ask the resident to remove their shoes. Help them stand on the scale. Make sure they are not holding anything.

6. _____ Have the resident stand up straight, with their arms by their side and their eyes looking forward. Slowly lower the height measurement bar to the top of their head. Record their height in feet and inches.

7. _____ Measure the resident's weight by moving the weights to the right until the balance needle is centered. **Note:** *If the weight is 5 pounds or more different from the previous measurement, weigh the resident again before reporting it to the charge nurse. If the resident is wearing a cast or brace when they are weighed, also report this to the nurse.*

8. _____ Help the resident off the scale.

9. _____ Record the resident's height and weight on the worksheet and report the findings to the charge nurse. Example of charting: Height: 5 feet 6 inches, Weight: 135 lbs

Note: *Your facility may have special scales for weighing residents while they are in a wheelchair or confined to bed. Follow your facility's policy and the manufacturer's instructions for using different scales.*

PROCEDURE 14-1 – MAKING AN UNOCCUPIED BED

1. _____ Look for any belongings in the bed. Residents may fall asleep with personal belongings under their pillow or elsewhere in the bed.

2. _____ Lower the head of the bed and raise the whole bed to a comfortable position (usually about hip level).

3. _____ Remove the spread and any blankets, and fold them on the chair.

4. _____ Remove soiled linen, including the pillowcase. Loosen sheets from under the mattress and carefully roll them into a ball, keeping the soiled side inside the ball and away from your body. (This keeps the cleaner side close to you. Rolling linens prevents the spread of organisms from dirty linens.) Put the sheets in the laundry bag.

5. ____ Check the mattress for any soiling or wetness. Wash and dry it with paper towels if necessary. Change the mattress pad if it is soiled or scheduled for change.
6. ____ If you are using a fitted sheet (shaped to the mattress by elastic edging), follow these steps:
Starting at the top corner of the mattress, wrap the edge of the mattress with the corner of the sheet, then go to the bottom of bed on the same side and wrap that edge. Do not shake the linen while unfolding it. (Shaking the linen raises dust and organisms.) Go to the opposite corner at the top of the bed and wrap that edge, and then wrap the last edge over the last corner. The sheet should fit the mattress snugly.
7. ____ If you are using a draw sheet, follow these steps: place it in the center of the bed so it covers the middle part of the bed. Tuck in the draw sheet on both sides. A draw sheet is often used for residents needing help with moving and positioning, or to keep bottom sheets clean and dry.
8. ____ If you are using a flat sheet follow these steps:
    a. ____ Unfold the bottom sheet lengthwise down the bed's center. Do not shake the linen while unfolding it. (Shaking linen raises dust and organisms.) Put the hem seams toward the mattress This keeps rough edges from touching the person.
    b. ____ Put the hem seams toward the mattress. This keeps rough edges from touching the person.
    c. ____ Slide the sheet so that the hem is even with the foot of the mattress. Keep the fold in the exact center of the bed from head to foot. (You want the extra length of sheet at the top to tuck it under the mattress).
    d. ____ Open the sheet from the fold so that the sheet covers the entire mattress and hangs evenly on both sides. Tuck the top hem in tightly under the mattresss at the head of the bed by lifting the head of the mattress and sliding the sheet under the mattress. Make a mitred corner (also called a hospital corner):
        i. ____ Face the side of the bed.
        ii. ____ With one hand, pick up the top of the sheet hanging down the side of the bed, and lay it on top of the bed so that it looks like a triangle.
        iii. ____ Tuck the remaining sheet under the mattress.
        iv. ____ Drop the section of sheet from on top of the bed over the side of the bed, and tuck it in.
    e. ____ Tuck the remaining sheet under the mattress neatly, starting from the mitered corner down to the foot of the mattress
    f. ____ If a draw sheet is used, open it up and place it in the center of the bed so it covers the middle part of the bed. Tuck in the draw sheet on the side you are working on. A draw sheet is often used for residents needing help with moving and positioning, or sometimes to keep bottom sheets clean and dry. You may also put any needed disposable incontinence pads over the draw sheet.
Continue with the top sheet:
9. ____ Place the top sheet on the bed. The wide hem should be even with the head of the mattress, with the seam on the outside. When you fold the hem over, the smooth side will be next to the resident's skin, preventing irritation from any rough edges. The excess sheet will be over the foot of the bed.
10. ____ Open the sheet from the fold so that the sheet covers the entire mattress and hangs evenly on both sides.
11. ____ Place the spread on top of the sheet in the same manner. Make sure the sheet does not hang below the spread on the sides.
12. ____ Tuck in the sheet and spread at the foot, making a mitered corner on the bottom end (Step 8d above).
13. ____ Smooth the sheet and spread from the bottom to the top of the bed, and fold down the top hem of the sheet over the spread.
14.   a. ____ Move to the other side of the bed and finish in the same way, starting with the bottom sheet and finishing with the top sheet and spread.
    b. ____ Pull the bottom sheet tight before each tuck to remove wrinkles. (Tuck in the draw sheet tightly if used.)
15. ____ Place a clean case on the pillow.
    a. ____ Hold the center of the closed end of the pillow case with your hand and turn it inside out over your hand;
    b. ____ Then grab the pillow with your hand inside the pillowcase and slide the case over the pillow. Make sure the corners of the pillow fit into the corners of the case.
    c. ____ Place the pillow(s) at the head of the bed, and fold the spread over them.
16. ____ Put the blanket at the foot of the bed or in the closet if a resident prefers.
17. ____ Return the bed to low position.

PROCEDURE 14-2 – MAKING AN OCCUPIED BED

1. ____ Lower the head of the bed, and remove the pillow from under the resident's head. (Do this only if the resident is comfortable in a completely flat position.)

2. ____ Remove the spread and any blankets, and place them folded on the chair.

3. ____ Loosen the top and bottom sheets from under the mattress. **Note:** *Side rails may be used for support in moving. If there is any risk that the resident could be injured by hitting the side rail, do not use it. Have another nurse assistant on the opposite side to support the resident if there is any risk of injury; make sure this person is ready to help before you begin.*

4. ____ Help the resident roll over on their side toward you. Raise the side rail and ask them to hold onto it for support. Go to the other side of the bed. Be sure the resident stays covered throughout the procedure.

5. ____ Check for any belongings in the bed.

6. ____ Roll lengthwise (top to bottom) the bottom soiled sheet from the side of the mattress to the center of the bed close to the resident's body. (If the linen is wet or very damp, place a barrier like a plastic-covered padding over the sheet.) Change the mattress pad if it is soiled or scheduled for changing.

7. ____ If you are using a fitted sheet (shaped to the mattress by elastic edging), follow these steps: Starting at the top corner of the mattress, wrap the edge of the mattress with the corner of the sheet; then go to the bottom of the bed on the same side and wrap the edge. Be sure half the mattress is covered and the sheet is tucked close to the resident.

8. ____ If you are using a draw sheet follow these steps: Place it in the center of the bed so it covers the middle part of the bed and is tucked close to the resident. Tuck in the draw sheet on the side you are working. A draw sheet is often used for residents needing help with moving and positioning, or sometimes to keep bottom sheets clean and dry. You may also put any needed disposable incontinence pads over the draw sheet.

9. ____ If you are using a flat sheet follow these steps:
   a. ____ Unfold the bottom sheet lengthwise, centered on the bed. Do not shake the linen while unfolding. (Shaking the linen raises dust and organisms.) Be sure the hem seams face the mattress. (This prevents any rough edges from touching the resident.)
   b. ____ Slide the sheet so that the hem is even with the foot of the mattress. Be sure to keep the fold in the exact center of the bed from head to foot. (You want the extra length of sheet at the top so that you can tuck it under the mattress.)
   c. ____ Open the sheet and fan-fold it lengthwise so that one half of the sheet is next to the rolled dirty sheet.
   d. ____ Tuck the top hem in tightly under the mattress at the head of the bed by lifting the mattress edge and sliding the sheet under it. Make a mitered corner:
      i. ____ Face the side of the bed.
      ii. ____ With one hand, pick up the top of the sheet hanging down the side of the bed, and lay it on top of the bed so it looks like a triangle.
      iii. ____ Tuck the remaining sheet under the mattress.
      iv. ____ Drop the section of sheet that is lying on top of the bed over the side of the bed, and tuck it in.
   e. ____ Tuck the remaining sheet under the mattress neatly, starting with the mitered corner down to the foot of the mattress.
   f. ____ If you are using a draw sheet, place it in the center of the bed so it covers the middle part of the bed. Fan-fold the excess and tuck it in with the sheet. Tuck in the draw sheet. A draw sheet is often used for residents needing help with moving and positioning, or sometimes to keep bottom sheets clean and dry.

Continue with the next steps:

10. ____ Flatten the rolled or fan-folded sheets and help the resident roll over the linen toward you, using the procedure for turning them (see Chapter 15, Moving and Positioning). Don't forget first to tell the resident that the roll of linen is behind them. **Note:** *Side rails may be used for support in moving. If there is any risk that the resident could be injured by the use of the rail, do not use it. Put up the side rail and ask the resident to hold onto it for support.*

11. ____ Go to the opposite side of the bed, lower the side rail, and remove the dirty bottom sheet. **Note:** *Never leave the resident unattended to take away dirty laundry. Put the dirty sheets in the laundry bag (if it is in the room) or at the bottom of the bed between the mattress and footboard.*

12. ____ Pull the clean linen toward you until it is completely unfolded, and tuck the sheets in tightly the same way as you did on the other side. Tuck in the draw sheet if used.

13. ____ Help the resident roll back to the center of the bed.

14. ____ Place the top sheet on the bed over the sheet covering the resident. Open the sheet from the fold so that the sheet hangs evenly on

each side of the bed. The wide hem should be at the top with the seam on the outside. When you fold the hem over, the smooth side will be next to the resident's skin, preventing any rough edges from touching them. The excess sheet is over the foot of the bed.

15. ____ Ask the resident to hold onto the clean sheet, then carefully remove the dirty top sheet by placing your hand under the clean top sheet and rolling the dirty sheet down toward the foot of the bed. Remove it and put it with the other dirty linen.

16 ____ Place the spread on top of the sheet in the same way you did the top sheet. Make sure the sheet does not hang below the spread on the sides.

17. ____ Tuck in the sheet and spread at the foot of the bed, and make a mitered corner at the bottom ends:
    a. ____ Face the side of the bed.
    b. ____ With one hand, pick up the top sheet hanging down the side of the bed, and lay it on top of the bed so it looks like a triangle.
    c. ____ Tuck the remaining sheet under the mattress.
    d. ____ Drop the sheet lying on top of the bed over the side of the bed, and tuck it in.

18. ____ Smooth the sheet and spread from the bottom to the top of the bed, and fold down the top hem of the sheet over the top of the spread. Be sure the top linens are not so tight that they are pressing on the resident's feet. To be sure, make a toe pleat. This is done by pulling the top linen up to form a pleat.

19. ____ Remove the dirty pillowcase, and put a clean case on the pillow. Hold the center of the closed end of the pillow case with your hand, turn it inside out over your hand, and then grab the pillow with the hand inside the pillow case and slide the case over the pillow. Make sure the corners of the pillow fit into the corners of the case. Put the pillow under the resident's head.

PROCEDURE 15-1 – MOVING UP IN BED WHEN A RESIDENT CAN HELP

1. ____ Put the head of the bed flat if the resident can tolerate it. Move the pillows against the headboard. **Note:** *Placing a pillow against the headboard will prevent the resident from injuring their head when moving up in bed.*

2. ____ Help the resident bend their knees up and place their feet flat on the bed. Place one arm under the resident's upper back behind the shoulders and the other under their upper thighs.

3. ____ On the count of three, have the resident push down with their feet and lift up their buttocks (bridging) while you help move them toward the head of the bed. **Note:** *You may also try having the resident help by using the side rails. Remember to put the side rails down when done.*

PROCEDURE 15-2 – MOVING UP IN BED WHEN A RESIDENT IS UNABLE TO HELP (TWO NURSE ASSISTANTS)

1. ____ Call another staff person to assist you.

2. ____ Put the head of the bed flat if the resident can tolerate it. Remove the pillow and place it against the headboard.

3. ____ Help the resident to cross their hands over their chest.

4. ____ Roll the draw sheet up from the side toward the resident until you and your helper both have a tight grip on it with both hands. Keep your palms up if that gives you more strength for moving. **Note:** *You can put one knee on the bed to get as close to the resident as possible.*

5. ____ Count aloud to 3, and you and your helper lift the resident up to the head of the bed, using good body mechanics. You can do this in stages until the resident is in position. **Note:** *If the resident is able, ask them to lift their head off the bed during the move.*

6. ____ Unroll the draw sheet and tuck it in.

PROCEDURE 15-3 – MOVING TO THE SIDE OF THE BED WHEN A RESIDENT CAN HELP

1. ____ Stand on the side to which you plan to move the resident.

2. ____ Help the resident bend their knees up and place their feet on the bed.

3. ____ Help the resident to bridge (lift up their buttocks), and move their buttocks to the side of the bed.

4. ____ Help the resident move their legs over, and then their head and upper body, by sliding your arms under them and gliding them toward you if they need help.

5. ____ You can do this in stages to reach the desired position.

PROCEDURE 15-4 – MOVING TO THE SIDE OF THE BED WHEN A RESIDENT IS UNABLE TO HELP

1. _____ Stand on the side to which you plan to move the resident.
2. _____ Ask the resident to fold their arms across their chest or do this for them if needed.
3. _____ Slide both your hands under the resident's head, neck, and shoulders and glide them toward you on your arms.
4. _____ Slide your arms under the residents' hips and glide them toward you.
5. _____ Slide your arms under their legs and glide them toward you. **Note:** *Keep the resident in proper body alignment.*

PROCEDURE 15-5 – MOVING A RESIDENT TO THE SIDE OF THE BED USING A DRAW SHEET

1. _____ Call another staff person to help you.
2. _____ Help the resident place their arms across their chest.
3. _____ Both you and your helper roll up the draw sheet from the sides toward the resident until you both have a good tight grip with both hands. (If the linen is soiled, use a barrier to prevent contaminating your uniform.) **Note:** *The staff person who is moving the resident away may want to put one knee on the edge of the bed to prevent injury caused by reaching too far. This person also leads the count because they have the heaviest part of the move.*
4. _____ Count aloud to 3, and on 3 you both lift the resident to the side of the bed. You can do this in stages until the desired position is reached.
5. _____ Unroll the draw sheet and tuck it in.

PROCEDURE 15-6 – TURNING A RESIDENT FROM SUPINE TO SIDE-LYING FOR PERSONAL CARE

1. _____ Help the resident bend their knees up one at a time and place their feet flat on the bed.
2. _____ Place one hand on the resident's shoulder farther away from you and the other hand on the hip farther from you.
3. _____ On the count of 3, help the resident roll toward you. Continue personal care.
Note: *Some residents may be more comfortable guiding the turn by holding onto the side rails.*

PROCEDURE 15-7 – MOVING THE RESIDENT FROM SUPINE POSITION TO SITTING

In this procedure, the resident begins on their back.

1. _____ Help the resident roll onto their side facing you, or elevate the head of the bed.
2. _____ Reach under the resident's head and put your hand under their shoulder (using your arm closer to the head of the bed). The resident's head should be supported by and resting on your forearm.
3. _____ With your other hand, reach over and behind the resident's knee farther from you.
4. _____ Using your legs and arms to do the lifting, bring the resident's head and trunk up as you swing their legs down to the sitting position. Hold the resident's legs, letting their knees rest in the crook of your elbow. **Note:** *Your arm behind the resident's head and body must stay in contact with the resident once they are sitting up to prevent them from falling backward. Remember to stay directly in front of the resident so you can block them with your body if needed for safety.*
   Note: *If you need a second staff person to help you assist the resident to sit up, both of you stand on the same side. One of you lifts the resident's head and body, while the other lifts their legs.*
5. _____ Help the resident get comfortable in the sitting position.

Another option is to:

1. _____ Help the resident roll onto their side facing you, or elevate the head of the bed.
2. _____ Slide their feet over edge of the bed.
3. _____ Reach under the resident's head and put your hand under their shoulder (using your arm closer to the head of the bed). The resident's head should be supported by and resting on your forearm.
4. _____ Place your other hand on the resident's hip. As you help the resident sit up, place gentle but firm pressure on their hip (using leverage) and help raise the resident's head to a sitting position. **Note:** *Your arm behind the resident's head and body must stay in contact with the resident once they are sitting up to prevent them from falling backward. Remember to stay directly in front of the resident so you can block them with your body if needed for safety.*

PROCEDURE 15-8 – MOVING THE RESIDENT FROM SITTING TO SUPINE POSITION

Note: *Before moving a resident from sitting to the supine position, be sure they are centered in the bed with the backs of their knees against the mattress. Help them push down on the floor with their feet and down on the bed with their hands to move their body back onto the bed in a sitting position.*

1. _____ Place one hand behind the resident's shoulder, and let their head and neck rest on your forearm. Place your other hand under their knees, and let their legs rest in the crook of your elbow. Position your arms as if you were carrying someone in front of you.

2. _____ Use your legs to lift and breathe out as you help the resident lift their legs up onto the bed. Gently lower their trunk and head onto the bed. **Note:** *You might want to elevate the head of the bed before helping the resident into the supine position. Once they are in bed, you can lower the head of the bed.*

PROCEDURE 15-9 – POSITIONING A RESIDENT ON THEIR BACK

1. _____ First move the resident's trunk and lower body so that their spine is in a neutral position. Do the positioning from the top of the body to the bottom.

2. _____ Position the resident's head and neck: Place a pillow under the resident's head and neck extending to the top of their shoulders. Do not elevate their head too high. Keep it as close to even with the chest as possible or as is comfortable.

3. _____ Position the resident's arms. The backs of the shoulders and elbows are common places for pressure ulcers in residents who cannot change positions by themselves. Vary their arm positions to prevent this. Keep their arms straight and resting on the mattress away from their sides, or bend their arms slightly at the elbow with a pillow between the inner arm and their side so that their arm rests on the pillow and their hand on top of the abdomen. Always support the arms in two places when moving them, and move them gently.

4. _____ Position the resident's legs: The sides of the hips, the buttocks, the sacrum and coccyx (the tip of the spine at the buttocks, or "tail bone"), and the backs of the heels are common places for pressure ulcers. Position the resident's legs straight and slightly apart. Always support the legs in two places when moving them, and move them gently. For those residents who tend to keep their legs tightly together or crossed, you may place a pillow between the resident's legs.

Note: *If a resident has ulcers on the sides of the hips, place a towel roll along the hip between the hip and the mattress on the affected side. If a resident has redness or ulcers under their heels, support their legs with a pillow lengthwise to raise their heels from the bed, or put a towel roll under their legs just above the heels.*

Note: *Support casts, splints, or swollen arms or legs by placing them on a pillow lengthwise to support the hand or foot higher than the rest of their arm or leg.*

PROCEDURE 15-10 – POSITIONING A RESIDENT ON THEIR SIDE (SIDE-LYING POSITION)

1. _____ Stand on the side to which the resident will be turning.

2. _____ Help the resident to bend their knees up.

3. _____ Place one hand on the resident's shoulder farther from you and the other on the hip farther from you. On the count of 3, help the resident roll toward you. Position the resident comfortably with proper body alignment.

4. _____ Position the resident's head and neck. Place the pillow under their head so that their top ear is almost level with their top shoulder.

5. _____ Fold a pillow lengthwise and place it behind the resident's back. Gently push the top edge of the pillow under their side and hip.

6. _____ Position the resident's arms. Gently pull the bottom arm out from under the resident's body if it is not already in front of the body. Place a pillow diagonally under the top arm between the arm and the resident's side. Bend the top arm or the elbow and shoulder to rest the arm on the pillow.

7. _____ Position the resident's legs. Bend the top hip up and rotate it slightly forward. Place a pillow lengthwise between the resident's knees to separate their legs down to their ankles.

Note: *Depending on the resident's condition, you can modify any of these positions to prevent pressure ulcers and make the resident comfortable.*

PROCEDURE 15-11 – THE STAND PIVOT TRANSFER

1. _____ Stand in front of the resident.

2. _____ Place one of your legs between the resident's legs and the other close to the target you are moving toward, such as a chair. (This gives you better control over the speed and the direction of the movement.)

3. _____ Hold onto the guard belt at the resident's back, slightly to either side. If you are not using a guard belt, put your arms around the resident's waist.

4. _____ Ask or help the resident to push down on the bed with their hands, lean forward, and stand up. If they are not able to do this, you can

have them hold your waist during the transfer. Do not let the resident hold you around your neck, which could injure you.

5. ____ On the count of 3 help the resident stand by leaning your body back and up, thereby bringing the resident's body forward. Ask them to lean forward and stand up.

6. ____ Once the resident is standing, keep your back neutral and body facing forward, and pivot (turn on your feet or take small steps) to turn them until the backs of their knees are against the chair.

7. ____ Ask the resident to reach back for the arm of the chair with one or both hands if possible.

8. ____ Help the resident bend their knees and sit.

9. ____ Once the resident is sitting, ask or help them to push back in the chair by pushing down with their feet on the floor and their arms on the armrests.

PROCEDURE 15-12 —ASSISTED TRANSFER WITH AN ASSISTIVE DEVICE (ONE PERSON)

1. ____ Once the resident is sitting on the side of the bed without difficulty, place the assistive device in their hand (cane) or in front of them (walker).

2. ____ Stand to the side of the resident on the side opposite the device.

3. ____ Ask or help the resident to push down on the bed with their hands and stand on the count of 3. You can help them by pulling up and forward on the back of the guard belt with one hand while pushing down on the walker or cane to keep it stable while the resident stands. Encourage a resident using a walker to stand before grabbing onto the assistive device.

4. ____ For residents using a walker, after they are standing, help them put both hands on the walker. **Note:** *Have the resident stand for a few minutes before trying to move, especially if they are dizzy.*

5. ____ Help the resident move toward the chair. Guide them with statements like these: "Turn, turn, take a step toward me, now back up."

6. ____ Help the resident back up to the chair. Ask if they can feel the chair against the back of their legs. Explain that they should not sit until they feel this.

7. ____ When the resident is in front of the chair, ask him them to reach back and put one hand on the armrest.

8. ____ Help the resident reach back with the other hand for the arm of the chair and slowly sit down.

PROCEDURE 15-13 – TRANSFERRING A RESIDENT FROM A CHAIR TO A BED, COMMODE, OR TOILET

1. ____ Position the chair with the resident's stronger side closer to the bed, commode, or toilet.

2. ____ If the resident is in a wheelchair, ask them to move their feet off the footrests. Raise up the footrests.

3. ____ Ask the resident to slide forward to the edge of the chair. This is often difficult, and the resident may need help.

4. ____ Use either the stand pivot or assistive device transfer procedure in reverse to move the resident from the chair and into bed.

PROCEDURE 15-14 – MOVING A RESIDENT WITH A MECHANICAL LIFT

1. ____ Adjust the head of the bed as flat as possible if the resident can tolerate it. To put the sling under the resident, first turn the resident toward you. Help the resident move toward you while your helper on the other side of the bed pushes the fan-folded sling under the resident as far as possible. Then help the resident back and toward the other side and pull the sling under them. **Note:** *The sling should be placed from under the resident's shoulders to the back of the knees. Have the same amount of sling material on both sides of the resident so that the resident is centered.*

2. ____ Place the lift frame facing the bed with its legs under the bed. Lock the wheels on the base.

3. ____ Elevate the head of the bed so the resident is partially sitting up.

4. ____ Attach the sling to the lift following the manufacturer's directions.

5. ____ Ask the resident to cross their arms over their chest before operating the lift. **Note:** *If a resident cannot keep their hands in their lap or across their chest, try having them hold onto an object on their lap.*

6. ____ Follow the manufacturer's directions to raise the resident up to a sitting position with the lift. While you operate the lift, your helper should help you guide the resident. **Note** *Repeatedly ask the resident if they are OK. Reassure the resident because this can be a frightening experience, especially the first time.*

7. ____ Once the resident is sitting, keep raising the lift until they are 6 to 12 inches over the bed and chair height.

8. ____ Unlock the swivel, if the lift has one, or use the steering handle to move the resident directly over the chair. You may need to guide the resident's legs.

9. ____ Tell the resident that you are now going to lower them slowly into the chair. Your helper guides the resident into the chair by moving the sling. Press the release button to slowly lower them down.
10. ____ Once the resident is securely in the chair, unhook the sling and remove the lift frame.
11. ____ Position the resident in the chair, leaving the sling under them (unless the sling is removable) until it is time to return to bed. Pull the metal bars of the sling out so that the resident does not lean against or sit on them.

PROCEDURE 15-15 – MOVING A RESIDENT UP IN A CHAIR
Note: *These steps are for moving a resident up in the chair after a transfer procedure to the chair. You need a helper for this procedure.*
1. ____ Place the guard belt on the resident.
2. ____ Standing on both sides of the resident, each of you grasps the guard belt with one hand and puts the other hand under the resident's knees. Ask the resident to cross their arms in front of their chest.
3. ____ On the count of 3, breathe out and lift the resident back in the chair. Be sure to use good body mechanics.

PROCEDURE 15-16 – RETURNING A RESIDENT TO BED USING A MECHANICAL LIFT
The process for returning a resident to bed reverses the steps for transferring a resident from the bed.
1. ____ Position the lift facing the chair.
2. ____ Attach the sling to the lift following the manufacturer's directions.
3. ____ Crank (or raise) the resident up with the lift. Your helper guides the resident by holding the sling.
4. ____ Swing the frame of the lift over the bed and slowly lower the resident down onto the bed.
5. ____ Unless the resident will spend only a short time in bed, roll them from side to side to remove the sling. (The sling could cause skin irritation if left under the resident.)
6. ____ Position the resident as preferred.

PROCEDURE 16-1 – COMPLETE BED BATH
Note: *Before beginning the bath, remove the resident's blanket and bedspread and put them on a clean surface. Put a bath blanket over the top sheet and then pull down the top sheet to the foot of the bed, leaving the bath blanket covering the resident. Expose only the part of the resident's body you are washing. This gives the person privacy and prevents them from becoming cold. Remove their clothing also under the bath blanket. The best position for the resident is flat in bed, if they can tolerate it. Fill the water basin halfway with water that is warm to your touch. Test the water with your bare hand– not with gloves on. The water temperature should be 98.6 F to 103 F. You can use a thermometer if one is available, or test the water temperature with the inside of your wrist, and then have the resident feel the water to be sure it is comfortable. Wash, rinse, dry, and inspect each body part. Be gentle. Start by making a bath mitt.*
Making a Bath Mitt: Make a bath mitt with the washcloth. The mitt provides a soft surface for the person's skin and is easier to use than an unfolded washcloth. The edges of an unfolded washcloth may get cold and make the resident uncomfortable.
1. ____ After wringing out the wet washcloth, put your hand in the center of the washcloth.
2. ____ Fold the side of the washcloth over from your little finger, and hold the fold with your thumb.
3. ____ Fold the remaining cloth over and hold it firmly with your thumb.
4. ____ Fold the top edge of the cloth down and tuck it into your palm. Hold it with your thumb.
5. ____ The mitt is now ready to use. Rinse the cloth and refold the mitt as needed during the bath.
Giving a Complete Bed Bath
1. ____ Begin with the resident's eyes, using only water–no soap. Start with the eye that is farther from you. With one corner of the washcloth, wash from the inner corner of the eye outward toward the ear. Clean away any crusting that may be stuck to the lower part of the eye. Use another corner of the washcloth to wash the near eye. Be sure to move the washcloth from the inner corner of the eye outward.
2. ____ Wash the resident's face. Some residents prefer not to use soap on their face. If so, use water only. Rinse, dry, and inspect the area. **Note:** *To wash with soap, wet the washcloth and apply a small amount of soap on it. Be sure to rinse the soap off. When you dry the resident's skin, pat it dry, being careful not to rub too hard.*
3. ____ Wash the resident's ears and neck. Rinse, dry, and inspect the area. **Note:** *When washing the resident's ears, wash behind the ear as well as inside. Wring out the wash cloth so that excess water does not enter the ear canal.*
4. ____ Wash the arms, underarm areas, and hands. Expose only the areas to be washed. Use a bath blanket to cover the resident. Use soap sparingly. (Remember: soap dries the skin.) Wash the side away from you first, then the side near you, so that you are moving from a

clean area to a dirty area, unless you feel you have to stretch too far and might injure yourself. (If so, wash one side of the resident's body, then move to the other side and wash it.) Rinse, dry, and inspect the area.

5. _____ Fold the bath blanket down and cover the resident's chest with a towel. Wash the chest and abdomen down as far as the pubic area. Rinse, dry, and inspect the area. Pay particular attention to the skin under a female resident's breasts and or any skin folds on the chest and abdomen. These are common areas for skin irritation and breakdowns. Note any redness, odor, or skin breakdown. Cover the chest with the bath blanket.

6. _____ Expose one leg, thigh, and foot. Cover the exposed leg with a towel. Wash the legs and feet. Don't forget to wash between the toes. Rinse, dry, and inspect the area. Check between the toes for any redness, irritation, or cracking of the skin. Note any swelling of the feet and legs. **Note:** *Change the water at this time or at any time during the bath if the water gets too cold, soapy, or dirty. (Using the same water after foot washing could potentially spread a foot fungus.) Cover up the resident before leaving to change the water.* Cover up the resident before leaving to change the water.

7. _____ Help the resident to turn to one side (see procedures for moving residents in Chapter 16). Keep the resident covered with a bath blanket.

8. _____ Expose the resident's back and buttocks. Wash the resident's back and buttocks. Rinse, dry, and inspect the area.

9. _____ Give the resident a back rub. Rub a small amount of lotion into your palms. Starting at the resident's lower back, gently move your hands up toward the shoulders, then downward to the lower back. Give the back rub for at least 3 minutes. Back rubs are comforting and relaxing and stimulate circulation, helping prevent skin breakdown. **Note:** *You may also give a back rub on request or as part of p.m. care.*

10. _____ Help the resident move back onto their back.

11. _____ Give perineal care (wash the genital and anal area of the body), as described below. **Note:** *After the back rub and before perineal care, put a plastic-covered pad under the resident to absorb water used to wash the perineal area, and put on a new pair of gloves. You can also use a bedpan for this. The bedpan allows a good view of the perineal area because it raises the resident's pelvis and lets you use more water for washing and rinsing. Since it might be uncomfortable for a resident, ask first. Sometimes you can use a fracture pan or a folded towel under the buttocks to raise the pelvis. Remember these guidelines:*
   • *Always change the water before perineal care.*
   • *Always change the washcloth and towel.*
   • *Always wear gloves when giving perineal care.*
   Note: *Perineal care is described here as part of a complete bed bath. If you do it separately, perform preparation and completion steps before and after the perineal care.*

12. _____ Help the resident get dressed.

Perineal Care for Female Residents

1. _____ Help the resident onto the bedpan or pad.

2. _____ Put on gloves.

3. _____ Drape the resident by folding back the bath blanket to expose only her legs and perineal area. Ask the resident to bend her knees.

4. _____ Have the resident check the water temperature to ensure that it is not too warm.

5. _____ Apply soap to a wet washcloth.

6. _____ Wash the pubic area with a downward stroke from the front to the back on each side of the labia. Make sure to use a clean area of the washcloth with each stroke.

7. _____ Wash downward in the middle over the urethra and vaginal opening. Always wash downward toward the anus with a clean area of the cloth to prevent the spread of infection.

8. _____ Using a second clean washcloth, rinse the soap from the pubic area using the same technique. Wipe front to back using a clean area of the cloth with each stroke.

9. _____ Dry the pubic area with a towel, and inspect the area for any redness, swelling, odor, drainage, or areas of irritation.

10. _____ After washing the genitals, turn the resident onto their side and then wash and rinse the anal area moving with upward strokes toward the back. Make sure to use a clean area of the cloth for each stroke.

11. _____ Dry with a clean towel.

12. _____ Reposition the resident for comfort.

Perineal Care for Male Residents

1. _____ Put on gloves.

2. ____ Drape the resident to expose only his legs and perineal area by folding back the bath blanket.

3. ____ Wash the penis from the urethral opening or tip of the penis toward the base of the penis, and then wash the scrotum. Take care to wash, rinse, and dry between any skin folds. Pull back the foreskin on uncircumcised males and clean under it. Return the foreskin. Check for any redness, swelling, or areas of irritation.

4. ____ Help the resident turn onto his side. Wash, rinse, and dry the anal area well, moving upward toward the back.

PROCEDURE 16-2 – TUB BATH

1. ____ Assist the resident to the tub room with all supplies. **Note:** *Some facilities may use chairs on wheels that may be taken to the resident's room. If you use this chair to bring the resident to the tub room, make sure that they are properly dressed and draped to protect their privacy and use the safety straps if needed and available.*

2. ____ Help the resident sit on the chair. Fill the tub halfway with warm water.

3. ____ Remember, always turn the hot water off first. **Note:** *The tub water should be in the range of 98.6 F to 103 F. Use a thermometer if available, or test the water temperature with the inside of your wrist, and then have the resident feel it with their hand or foot. The resident's doctor may order special medication to be added to the bath water, such as bran, oatmeal, starch, sodium bicarbonate, Epsom salts, pine products, sulfa, potassium permanganate, or salt. Always check with the charge nurse about the proper use of any of these substances.*

4. ____ Help the resident remove their clothing.

5. ____ Check that the bath mat is in place. Help the resident into the tub.

6. ____ Help with bathing as needed. (Put gloves on if you will be assisting with perineal care.) **Note:** *Never leave the resident alone while bathing in a tub. Always encourage residents to use safety rails. Be sure to check the water temperature during the tub bath to be sure it has not cooled down. Add hot water as needed.*

7. ____ Place a clean towel on the seat of the chair.

8. ____ Help the resident out of the tub. Encourage them to use safety rails. Cover them with a bath blanket

9. ____ Help the resident with drying, applying personal hygiene products, and dressing. **Note:** *You may give them a back rub before dressing, if the resident desires.*

10. ____ Help the resident back to their room. Bring any of their personal hygiene products back to their room.

PROCEDURE 16-3 – SHOWER

1. ____ Help the resident to the shower room with all necessary supplies.

2. ____ Help the resident sit on the chair, using safety straps if needed and available.

3. ____ Turn on the shower with warm water. Test the water on the inside of your wrist and have the resident feel it with their hand or foot. Adjust the temperature as needed.

4. ____ Help the resident remove their clothing.

5. ____ Help the resident into the shower. Encourage them to use the safety rails. **Note:** *Most facilities have shower chairs that lock in place. If the resident needs to shower sitting down, be sure the shower chair is locked before they sit down.*

6. ____ Help the resident with showering as needed. (Wear gloves if you help with perineal care.) Encourage the resident to participate in bathing as much as possible. Give help and verbal cueing as needed. Wash from head to toe. Rinse the washcloth as needed. **Note:** *Bathing is a good time to observe the resident's skin for any skin conditions, to conduct range-of-motion exercises, and to engage in conversation with the resident. These acts add restorative care into the resident's daily routine.*
Note: *If the resident is not shampooing, use a shower cap to prevent their hair from getting wet.*

7. ____ Place a dry towel on the chair outside the shower.

8. ____ Help the resident out of the shower and onto the covered chair. Cover the resident with a bath blanket.

9. ____ Turn off the shower. Turn the hot water off first to prevent a burn.

10. ____ Help the resident dry off, use personal hygiene products, and get dressed. **Note:** *You may give a back rub at this point if desired.*

11. ____ Help the resident back to their room. Bring their personal hygiene products back to the room and put them away.

PROCEDURE 16-4 – WHIRLPOOL BATH

1. ____ Help the resident to the whirlpool room with all supplies.

2. _____ Help the resident sit on a chair.
3. _____ Turn on the water in the whirlpool following the facility's procedure. The water temperature should be 98.6 F to 103 F. Test the water temperature on the inside of your wrist, and have the resident feel it with their hand or foot. Adjust the temperature as needed.
4. _____ Help the resident remove their clothing.
5. _____ Help the resident into the whirlpool bath. Encourage use of safety rails. **Note:** *Follow the manufacturer's and facility's guidelines. If you use a mechanical lift, be sure you know how to use it properly.*
6. _____ Help the resident bathe. Encourage the resident to participate in bathing as much as possible. Give help and verbal cueing as needed. Wash from head to toe. Rinse the wash cloth as needed. Wear gloves if you help with perineal care. Never leave the resident unattended. **Note:** *If the resident has a wound dressing, ask the nurse to remove it before the bath and apply a clean one afterward. If the doctor has ordered an antiseptic solution in the whirlpool bath, the nurse will add the solution or give you specific instructions.*
7. _____ Place a dry towel on the chair.
8. _____ Help the resident out of the whirlpool bath and onto the covered chair. Encourage them to use the safety rails. Cover them with a bath blanket.
9. _____ Help the resident dry off, apply personal hygiene products, and get dressed. **Note:** *You may give them a back rub at this point if desired.*
10. _____ Help the resident back to their room.

PROCEDURE 16-5 – SHAMPOOING AND CONDITIONING

1. _____ Help the resident into a chair.
2. _____ Comb or brush out any tangles before shampooing.
3. _____ Turn on the water to a warm temperature, no more than 103° F. Test the water temperature on the inside of your wrist, and have the resident feel it with their hand.
4. _____ Help the resident take off their clothes for showering or tub bathing. Wash the resident's hair as the resident prefers (some residents want it done first, and some last). If a resident is shampooing at the sink, put the back of the chair against the front of the sink. Pad the rim of the sink with a towel. Position the resident for the method you are using: upright in a shower chair, flat in bed with pillows placed under their shoulders, or tilted in shampoo chair. Protect their clothes with a towel draped over the shoulders. If you are shampooing in bed, you need a shampoo trough, basin, or pail, and a waterproof bed protector.
5. _____ Wet the hair entirely. Place a face cloth over the resident's eyes to prevent shampoo from getting into the resident's eyes.
6. _____ Pour a small amount of shampoo into your palm and apply it to the resident's wet hair. Massage the shampoo gently throughout hair and scalp.
7. _____ Rinse the hair well with warm water.
8. _____ Apply conditioner, if used.
9. _____ Rinse the hair well with warm water.
10. _____ Help the resident out of the shower or tub into the chair. Cover them with a bath blanket. Wrap a towel around their hair. Help them dry off and get dressed. If the resident is in bed, help them wipe their face with the towel used to protect their eyes. Remove the trough or basin from beneath the resident's head. Remove the waterproof sheet from under their head and shoulders. Change the linen as necessary. Position the resident with the head of the bed up.
11. _____ Dry their hair thoroughly and quickly to prevent chilling. Use a hair dryer on a low setting if available.
12. _____ Style the resident's hair as they like it. Check for any flaking, reddened areas, or other scalp problems. **Note:** *Some residents use special shampoos or conditioners, often with medicine the doctor orders for a specific condition. Ask the nurse for instructions and read the labels carefully before using them.*
13. _____ Help the resident back to their room.

PROCEDURE 16-6 – BRUSHING AND FLOSSING

Note: *You can help residents with brushing and flossing at the bedside table or the resident's sink, as they prefer.*

1. _____ Apply a small amount of toothpaste to the wet toothbrush and set it aside. Mix water and mouthwash in a cup. A solution of half water, half mouthwash is best. Set this aside. Mouthwash is strong and could be harmful to sensitive gums.
2. _____ Break off or least 18 inches of floss. Set this aside.
3. _____ Put on gloves. **Note:** *If you know that the resident's gums bleed, talk with the charge nurse about other personal protective equipment you may need, like protective eye wear and face mask.*

4. ____ Put a towel over the resident's chest to protect their clothing.
5. ____ Give the resident a small amount of mouthwash solution to swish around in their mouth to rinse it. Place the emesis basin under the resident's chin so they can spit out the solution.
6. ____ Brush the resident's upper teeth and gums first, moving the brush from the gums to the teeth downward. Then brush the lower teeth and gums moving again from the gums to the teeth upward. Be sure to brush the back of the teeth. Inspect the teeth and gums while brushing.
7. ____ Brush the tongue gently.
8. ____ Help the resident rinse their mouth with a little mouthwash solution.
9. ____ Wrap the ends of the floss around your middle fingers of each hand to get a good grip. Gently insert the floss between each tooth and the next. Move the floss to the gum line and down between the teeth. Wrap the floss around your fingertips to keep using a clean section as you move from tooth to tooth.
10. ____ Have the resident rinse their mouth thoroughly.
11. ____ Dry any solution around the resident's mouth or chin.

PROCEDURE 16-7 – CARING FOR DENTURES
1. ____ Put on gloves.
2. ____ Ask the resident to remove their dentures and place them in the denture cup. If the resident cannot remove their own dentures, follow these steps.
   a. ____ Place a towel over the resident's chest.
   b. ____ Rinse the resident's mouth with mouthwash solution to moisten it. Ask them to swish the solution around, and put the emesis basin under their chin so the resident can spit out the solution.
   c. ____ Remove the upper denture using a paper towel for a better grip. Loosen the denture by gently rocking it back and forth to help break the seal. Put it in the denture cup.
   d. ____ Remove lower denture using a paper towel for better grip. Loosen it by gently rocking it back and forth. Put it in the denture cup.
3. ____ Rinse the resident's mouth with mouthwash solution.
4. ____ If the resident cannot rinse, use a swab moistened with water and mouthwash to clean the whole mouth, including the tongue and gums.
5. ____ Explain that you will clean the dentures and then return them.
6. ____ Take the denture cup with dentures, toothbrush, and toothpaste to the resident's bathroom.
7. ____ Put toothpaste on the toothbrush.
8. ____ Turn on cool water (hot water can damage dentures), put a small towel or face cloth on the bottom of the sink, and fill the sink halfway. (This helps prevent dentures from breaking if they slip from your hands.)
9. ____ Hold the dentures over the sink and brush all surfaces.
10. ____ Rinse the dentures with cool water.
11. ____ Return the dentures to the denture cup.
12. ____ If the resident uses denture adhesive, apply it to the dentures before putting them back in their mouth. If the resident does not want the dentures put back at this time, store them safely. Put them in a denture cup labeled with the resident's name and half filled with cool water.

Note: *Inspect the resident's mouth for bleeding, sores, a dry, coated tongue, and mouth odor. Report any changes to the nurse. If the resident has a partial plate with only a few artificial teeth, handle it the same way as a complete set of dentures. Be careful when you remove the partial plate, which has wires that support the teeth in place.*

PROCEDURE 16-8 – MOUTH CARE FOR COMATOSE RESIDENTS
1. ____ Gently turn the resident's head toward you and elevate the head of the bed (if they can tolerate it) to prevent aspiration.
2. ____ Put a towel over the resident's chest to protect their clothing.
3. ____ Put on gloves.
4. ____ Gently open the resident's mouth and inspect the mouth, teeth, gums, and tongue for changes or signs of injury: bleeding sores, loose or broken teeth, dry coated tongue, or mouth odor. Using a toothette dipped in mouthwash, clean the inside of the mouth (gums, tongue, teeth, roof of the mouth, and insides of the cheeks). **Note:** *Tap excess mouthwash off the toothette. Excess fluid can drip back into their throat and potentially cause aspiration.*

5. ____ Using a corner of the towel draped over the resident's chest, dry any solution from around their mouth and chin.
6. ____ Dispose of toothettes as you use them into the plastic trash bag.
7. ____ Put protective jelly or lip balm on their lips to moisten them.

PROCEDURE 16-9 – SHAVING A MALE RESIDENT'S FACE
1. ____ Observe the resident's face for any moles, rashes, or cuts. Do not shave those areas, or use extra care.
2. ____ Place a towel over the resident's chest to protect their clothing.
3. ____ Put on gloves.
4. ____ Using a face cloth, wet the entire beard with warm water and apply shaving cream with your hands.
5. ____ When the beard is well lathered and softened, start shaving. Shave in the direction the beard grows. Hold the skin tight and smooth by pulling the skin upward with one hand and shaving with a downward stroke with your other hand. Use short, even strokes. Be particularly careful with the neck, chin, and upper lip. Use upward strokes for the neck, downward and slightly diagonal strokes for the chin, and very short downward strokes above the lip.
6. ____ Rinse the razor in warm water after each stroke.
7. ____ Wash and rinse the resident's face with the washcloth, dry his face, and apply aftershave lotion if he prefers.
8. ____ Give the resident a mirror to look at his face.
9. ____ Remove the towel from the resident's chest.

PROCEDURE 16-10 – SHAVING A FEMALE RESIDENT'S UNDERARMS
1. ____ Put the towel under the resident's shoulder on the side you are working from.
2. ____ Raise the resident's arm up along their ear to expose the underarm.
3. ____ Wash the area with warm water.
4. ____ Lather some soap and apply it over the area to be shaved.
5. ____ Carefully shave the area, moving the razor downward from the arm toward the chest.
6. ____ Rinse the soap away thoroughly and pat the area dry.
7. ____ Move the towel to under the opposite shoulder and repeat the steps above.

PROCEDURE 16-11 – SHAVING A FEMALE RESIDENT'S LEGS
1. ____ Place a towel under the resident's leg to be shaved.
2. ____ Wash the part of the leg to be shaved with warm water.
3. ____ Lather some soap or use shaving cream. Spread it over the entire area to be shaved.
4. ____ Carefully shave the area, moving the razor upward from the ankle to the knee. **Note:** *Ask the resident if she wants the area above her knee shaved.*
5. ____ Be sure to rinse the soap thoroughly and pat the area dry.
6. ____ Move the towel under the other leg and repeat the steps above.

PROCEDURE 16-12 – TRIMMING FACIAL HAIR
1. ____ Using safety scissors, carefully trim the facial hair. Be careful not to trim too close to the skin.
2. ____ Give the resident a mirror to look at her face.

PROCEDURE 16-13 – HAIR CARE
1. ____ Brush hair gently. If the resident's hair is long and tangled, remove tangles first with a comb. Start at the ends and work your way up to the scalp.
2. ____ Gently brush and style the hair to the resident's preference. Use any personal items they may request, such as hair spray, clips, or gel.
3. ____ Give the resident a mirror so they can see their hair.

PROCEDURE 16-14 – CARE OF FINGERNAILS

1. ____ Place the basin of warm water on the over-bed table.
2. ____ Ask the resident to soak their hands in the basin 3-5 minutes.
3. ____ Leaving one hand in the water, wash and rinse the resident's other hand. Dry the hand and place it on a dry towel.
4. ____ Clean under the nails with the orangewood stick.
5. ____ Repeat with the other hand.
6. ____ Inspect the resident's hands for cracks in the skin, unusual spots or discoloration, and rough areas.
7. ____ Trim the resident's fingernails using the nail clipper. Clip nails straight across. Shape and remove any rough edges using an emery board or nail file.
8. ____ Put lotion on the resident's hands and gently massage the hands from fingertips toward the wrists to stimulate circulation.
9. ____ Tell the nurse about any redness, irritation, broken skin, or loose skin.

PROCEDURE 16-15 – CARE OF TOENAILS

1. ____ To give foot care to a resident sitting in a chair, put a towel on the floor and the basin of water on the towel. **Note:** *Foot care can be done while a resident is in bed, usually during a bed bath. Put a towel on the bed and the basin on the towel. Ask the resident to flex their leg and soak one foot at a time.*
2. ____ Help the resident to remove their shoes and socks.
3. ____ Place the resident's feet in the basin of warm water.
4. ____ Soak the feet for 3-5 minutes.
5. ____ Clean under the toenails with the orangewood stick to remove any dirt. Scrub callused areas with a warm wash cloth.
6. ____ Wash, rinse, dry, and inspect the feet thoroughly. Report any redness, irritation, or cracked, broken, loose, dry, or discolored skin. Report any callused areas, corns, or loose or broken nails.
7. ____ Apply lotion to the tops of the feet, soles of the feet, and heels. Do not apply lotion between the toes.
8. ____ Help the resident put on clean stockings or socks and shoes.
9. ____ Tell the charge nurse if the resident needs toenail trimming.

PROCEDURE 16-16 – DRESSING A DEPENDENT RESIDENT

Note: *If a resident has a weak or paralyzed arm or has an IV in one arm, help them to put a shirt or dress sleeve on that arm first. With an IV, move the solution through the sleeve first and hang it on the pole. Gently guide the resident's arm through the sleeve, being careful not to dislodge the IV needle or tube. If the resident has an IV pump, call the nurse for assistance. Use this method also for a weak leg. Dress the weak side first.*

1. ____ Offer the resident a choice of clothing and then remove the resident's gown or pajamas. **Note:** *For privacy and to prevent chill, remove the top portion of the resident's gown or pajamas first. Help the resident dress on top with clean clothes, and then move to the bottom.*
2. ____ Help the resident put on their undershirt or bra, shirt or blouse, or dress.
3. ____ Help the resident put on underwear, stockings or socks, and pants or a skirt. Depending on the type of garment, follow these steps:
   To put on a garment that opens in the back:
   a. ____ Slide the garment onto the resident's arm and shoulder on the weaker side.
   b. ____ Slide the garment onto the arm and shoulder of the stronger side.
   c. ____ Bring the sides of the garment to the back.
   d. ____ Turn the resident toward you, and bring the side of the garments to the back.
   e. ____ Turn the resident away from you, and bring the other side of the garment to the resident's back.
   f. ____ Fasten the buttons, snaps, ties, or zipper.
   g. ____ Place the resident in the supine position.
   To put on a garment that opens in the front:
   a. ____ Slide the garment onto the resident's arm and shoulder on the weaker side.
   b. ____ Bring the resident to a sitting position, and bring the garment around the back. Lower the resident to the supine position.
   c. ____ Slide the garment onto the resident's arm and shoulder on the stronger side.
   d. ____ Fasten buttons, snaps, ties, or zipper.

To put on a pullover garment:

a. _____ Place the resident in the supine position.

b. _____ Bring the neck of the garment over the resident's head.

c. _____ Slide the arm and shoulder of the garment onto the resident's weaker side.

d. _____ Raise the resident to a semi-sitting position, bring the garment down over the their shoulder, and slide the arm and shoulder of the garment on the resident's stronger side. **Note:** *If the resident cannot assume a sitting position, turn the resident toward you and pull the garment down on the back. Then turn the resident to the other side, and slide their stronger arm and shoulder into the garment. Pull the garment down in the back.*

e. _____ Fasten the buttons, snaps, ties, or zipper.

To put on pants or slacks:

a. _____ Slide the pants over the resident's feet and up their legs.

b. _____ Ask the resident to raise their hips and buttocks off the bed.

c. _____ Bring the pants up over their buttocks and hips. **Note:** *If the resident cannot raise their buttocks and hips, turn them onto their stronger side. Then pull the pants up over their hips and buttocks on their weaker side. Turn the resident onto the other side and repeat the process.*

d. _____ Fasten the buttons, snaps, ties, or zipper.

4. _____ Help the resident put on socks, shoes, or non-skid slippers before they stand, so that they do not slip on the floor. When you put their shoes on in bed, put a pad on the bed to protect bedding.

5. _____ Help the resident stand so you can smooth out their clothing and fasten and neatly tuck in their shirt or blouse.

6. _____ Help them put on any accessories they want to wear.

7. _____ If a resident has a prosthesis or adaptive equipment (such as eyeglasses, dentures, hearing aid, or an artificial limb), help the resident to put the item on.

8. _____ Collect soiled garments, and place them in a hamper for the laundry according to the facility's procedure.

Note: *Residents are usually helped out of bed after dressing for the day.*

PROCEDURE 16-17 – UNDRESSING A DEPENDENT RESIDENT

Note: *This procedure is easier if the resident is sitting on the side of the bed.*

Note: *If a resident has a weak or paralyzed arm or an IV, remove clothing from other side first and then from the weak side or the side with the IV. If the resident has an IV, carefully guide the tubing and solution through the sleeve as the resident's arm moves.*

1. _____ Help the resident remove upper garments (shirt, dress, blouse, and undergarments).

2. _____ Help the resident put on the top half of their pajamas or nightgown.

3. _____ Help the resident remove their shoes or stockings and pants or skirt.

4. _____ If wearing pajamas, help them put on their bottoms.

5. _____ Help the resident into bed.

ASSISTING RESIDENTS WITH MEALS (CHAPTER 17)

1. _____ Prepare residents before the meal. Help them as needed with grooming, handwashing, and oral care. Residents should sit upright at a 90-degree angle, with their feet touching the floor.

2. _____ Help residents to the dining room or make them comfortable in their rooms. If possible, transfer the resident from a wheelchair to a dining room chair.

3. _____ Wash your hands.

4. _____ Position napkins and clothing protectors.

5. _____ Pass trays quickly to ensure cold foods stay cold and hot foods hot.

6. _____ Check tray cards: Make sure the name matches the person and the diet appears correct and complete. Check for any special feeding instructions.

7. _____ Put the plate on the table, open cartons, remove wrappings, cut meats, and season food as the resident prefers.

8. _____ While serving the meal, describe foods positively.

9. _____ Make sure each resident is close enough to the table to reach their food and silverware.

10. _____ Encourage residents to feed themselves as much as possible.

11.   Serve all residents at one table before moving to the next.
12.   Check with residents frequently to offer assistance or substitutes for foods they are not eating.
13.   Be sure each resident has enough time to finish their meal.
14.   Remove the tray and make sure each resident's hands and face are clean and that they are comfortable.

GENERAL FEEDING GUIDELINES FOR FEEDING MOST RESIDENTS (CHAPTER 17)

1.   Prepare each resident for the meal. Provide oral care, wash the resident's hands, and make the resident comfort- able. Check the resident's positioning. Elevate the head of the bed to at least 70 to 90 degrees. Cover the resident with a clothing protector or a large napkin. Remember to preserve the resident's dignity at all times. Make sure to check the tray card and ask the resident their name to ensure the accuracy of the meal being served.
2.   Take foods off the tray and put them on the table in front of the resident, and describe each one. Encourage residents to help themselves eat in any way possible, such as by holding their own cup.
3.   Use a spoon from which the resident can easily remove the food. Usually a teaspoon is better than a soup spoon. Fill the spoon no more than half full. Feed residents in a manner as close to normal as possible to preserve their dignity. Sit down next to the resident while feeding them. Speak softly to the resident, and maintain eye contact. Let the resident decide what to eat and in what order.
4.   Be aware of food temperatures. If the food seems too hot, give it time to cool. Do not mix foods together unless the resident requests this.
5.   Encourage the resident to eat more nutritious foods first. Save dessert until last if possible. Offer small bites, making sure the resident swallows each bite before offering another. Do not rush the resident. Offer liquids between bites to keep their mouth moist.
6.   Have a caring attitude.
7.   Encourage residents to eat all of their meal. As with all residents, offer to get a substitute if they are not eating or refuse some food.
8.   When the resident is finished eating, remove the clothing protector, any remaining food, and the tray.
9.   Give oral care.
10.   Report to the charge nurse any changes in the resident that occur with feeding, such as nausea, stomach ache, choking, or decreased appetite.

PROCEDURE 18-1 – HELPING A RESIDENT USE A BEDPAN

1.   Put on gloves. **Note:** *If you contaminate your gloves in any way during the procedure, you must change to a new pair of gloves.*
2.   Put a pad or cover on the surface where you will put the bedpan after it is used.
3.   Fold the bedspread and blanket down to the bottom of the bed, leaving the top sheet in place to cover the resident's lower legs. Help the resident lift their nightgown or remove pajama bottoms or underpants.
4.   Put a protective cover under the resident's buttocks to protect the bed linen.
5.   Ask the resident to bend both knees and lift their buttocks up while you slide the bedpan underneath them. Adjust it for the resident's comfort. Sometimes using powder or cornstarch on the bedpan prevents the resident's skin from sticking to it when the bedpan is removed. **Note:** *If the resident does not have the strength to lift their buttocks, ask or help them turn onto one side (as described in Chapter 15). Hold the bedpan flush against their buttocks and have the resident turn back onto the bedpan. (You may need help from another nurse assistant.)*
6.   Remove your gloves and dispose of them.
7.   Cover the resident with the top sheet for privacy.
8.   Elevate the head of the bed slowly until the resident is in a sitting position. (Remember: You are trying to create a normal setting.) Ask the resident if they are as comfortable as they can be. Change the position of the bedpan if needed to make them comfortable.
9.   Provide toilet paper and position the call light button so the resident can reach it. Tell them to call you when finished. If a resident cannot tell you they are finished, check on them every 5 minutes. Because a bedpan puts pressure on the skin, do not leave a resident on a bedpan longer than needed.

To help a resident from the bedpan:

10.   Put on gloves.
11.   Lower the head of the bed. Ask the resident to lift their buttocks up while you slide the bedpan out. If needed, help them roll onto one side while you hold the bedpan to prevent a spill. Move the bedpan to the covered surface.
12.   If needed, help with wiping the perineal area. Put the used toilet tissue in the bedpan. You may need to wash the perineal area for some residents. (Remember to wash, rinse, and dry thoroughly.) Wash or wipe from front to back. Remove and dispose of the protective

pad over the bed linen. **Note:** *Some facilities may have premoistened disposable washcloths for perineal care or use a commercial cleanser that is put in a bottle. You squeeze this solution from the bottle over the perineal area.*

13. ____ Remove your soiled gloves and put on clean gloves.
14. ____ Help the resident wash their hands. **Note:** *If perineal washing was necessary, change the water and use a fresh washcloth and towel for hand washing. Remove your gloves , dispose of them, and put on a new pair before proceeding.*
15. ____ Help the resident get dressed.
16. ____ Put the bedpan cover on the bedpan and dispose of the contents in the resident's toilet. Clean the bedpan and return it to the bedside table. Remove and dispose of the protective pad on which you put the bedpan. **Note:** *Most facilities have a water sprayer attached to the toilet for cleaning bedpans, urinals, etc. You will learn the procedure for emptying and cleaning equipment in your facility. When you clean the equipment, be careful not to splash the contents.*
17. ____ Remove and dispose of your gloves in the disposable trash bag, throw the trash bag away, and wash your hands.

PROCEDURE 18-2 – HELPING A MALE RESIDENT USE A URINAL

1. ____ Put on gloves. **Note:** *If you contaminate your gloves in any way during the procedure, you must change to a new pair of gloves.*
2. ____ Put a pad or cover on the surface where you will put the urinal after use. **Note:** *If the resident can stand beside the bed to use the urinal, help him to stand, and provide privacy. Put the call light button within reach so he can call you when finished; then continue with Steps 6-12.*

If a resident uses the urinal while in bed, follow these steps:

3. ____ Fold the bedspread and blanket down to the bottom of the bed, leaving the top sheet over the resident. Help the resident lower his bottom clothing.
4. ____ Place the urinal between the resident's legs at an angle to avoid urine spillage. Gently place the penis into the urinal.
5. ____ Take off your gloves and put them in a plastic trashbag. Cover the resident with the top sheet and give him the call light. Tell him to call you when he is done. Check in a few minutes if he does not call you.
6. ____ Put on new gloves.
7. ____ When the resident is finished, remove the urinal and place it on the covered surface.
8. ____ If needed, help the resident wipe off excess urine with toilet tissue. Dispose of tissue and your gloves in the plastic trash bag.
9. ____ Put on new gloves.
10. ____ Help the resident wash, rinse, and dry his hands.
11. ____ Empty the urinal, clean it, and replace it in the bedside table. **Note:** *most facilities have a water sprayer attached to the toilet for cleaning bedpans, urinals, etc. You will learn the procedure for emptying and cleaning equipment in your facility. When you clean the equipment, be careful not to splash the contents.*
12. ____ Remove and dispose of your gloves in the disposable trash bag, throw the trash bag away, and wash your hands.

PROCEDURE 18-3 – HELPING A RESIDENT USE A PORTABLE COMMODE

1. ____ Put on gloves. **Note:** *If you contaminate your gloves in any way during the procedure, you must change to a new pair of gloves.*
2. ____ Help the resident out of bed to a standing position (as described in Chapter 15, Moving and Positioning). Help pull down the resident's lower clothing. Help them sit on the commode positioned by the bed. **Note:** *Position the commode so it will not move when you help the resident out of bed. Put the commode against the wall or against the bedside table to keep it from moving.*
3. ____ Provide toilet paper and put the call light button within reach.
4. ____ If the resident needs help with wiping when finished:
   a. ____ Put on gloves.
   b. ____ Help with wiping, and throw the tissue into the commode or plastic trash bag.
   c. ____ Take off your gloves and put them in the plastic trash bag.
5. ____ Help the resident with their clothing and to get back into the bed or chair.
6. ____ Put on new gloves.
7. ____ Help the resident wash, rinse, and dry their hands.
8. ____ Remove the container from the commode and empty its contents into the toilet in the bathroom. **Note:** *Most facilities have a water sprayer attached to the toilet for cleaning bedpans, urinals, etc. You will learn the procedure for emptying and cleaning equipment in your facility. When you clean the equipment, be careful not to splash the contents.*

9. _____ Clean and dry the container and put it back in the commode.

10. _____ Remove and dispose of your gloves in the disposable trash bag, throw the trash bag away, and wash your hands.

PROCEDURE 18-4 – COLLECTING A URINALYSIS SPECIMEN

1. _____ Have the resident void or urinate into a bedpan, urinal (if male), or clean hat in the toilet.

2. _____ Put on gloves. **Note:** *If you contaminate your gloves in any way during the procedure, you must change to a new pair of gloves.*

3. _____ Pour about 60 cc of urine in the specimen container. Discard the urine left over by emptying it into the toilet.

4. _____ Write the resident's name, room number, and date and time you collected the specimen on the container's label.

5. _____ Place the specimen container in a biohazardous plastic bag and close it properly.

6. _____ Remove and dispose of your gloves in the disposable trash bag, throw the trash bag away, and wash your hands.

PROCEDURE 18-5 – COLLECTING A CLEAN-CATCH URINALYSIS SPECIMEN

1. _____ Put on gloves. **Note:** *If you contaminate your gloves in any way during the procedure, you must change to a new pair of gloves.*

2. _____ Clean the urethral opening.

   a. _____ For a female resident, use one wipe to clean one side of the labia, a second wipe to clean the other side of the labia, and a third wipe to clean down the middle. Always clean in single strokes from front to back. Use each wipe only once and then dispose of it.

   b. _____ Clean the penis following the procedure used for perineal care. For an uncircumcised male resident, pull back the foreskin of the penis to clean it.

3. _____ Have the resident begin to urinate and then stop if they can. Do not collect this first urine. **Note:** *If the resident cannot stop the flow of urine, you have to put the container under the stream before they finish to get enough urine.*

4. _____ Hold the specimen container under the urethra, ask the resident to begin voiding again, and collect the remainder of the specimen.

5. _____ Write the resident's name, room number, and the date and time you collected specimen on the specimen container.

6. _____ Place the specimen container in a plastic bag and close it.

7. _____ Remove and dispose of your gloves in the disposable trash bag, throw the trash bag away, and wash your hands after handling each specimen.

PROCEDURE 18-6 – COLLECTING A 24-HOUR URINE SPECIMEN

1. _____ Remind the resident not to throw out any urine. Place a sign in the bathroom to alert other staff or family. (Everyone involved needs to understand that if any urine is lost, the test may need to be restarted.) All urine must be collected in the same container.

2. _____ Always put on gloves before handling specimens.

3. _____ Discard the first voided urine of the day. At this time the collection period of 24 hours begins. (The test would be inaccurate if the first voided urine was not discarded, because it contains urine that collected in the bladder before the starting period.) During the collection period the resident should use a bedpan, commode, urinal, or collection hat on the toilet. Remind the resident to call you each time they urinate so that you can be sure all urine specimens are collected.

4. _____ Remove and dispose of your gloves in the disposable trash bag, throw the trash bag away, and wash your hands after handling each specimen.

When the 24 hours are up:

5. _____ Put on a new pair of gloves.

6. _____ Write the resident's name, room number, and the date and the collection time period on the specimen container.

7. _____ Place the specimen container in a biohazardous plastic bag and close it.

8. _____ Remove and dispose of your gloves in the disposable trash bag, throw the trash bag away, and wash your hands after handling each specimen.

PROCEDURE 18-7 – TESTING URINE FOR KETONES

1. _____ Put on gloves. **Note:** *If you contaminate your gloves in any way during the procedure, you must change to a new pair of gloves.*

2. _____ Have the resident void in the bedpan, urinal, or hat on a toilet.

3. _____ Either dip the end of the strip in the fresh urine or pass it through the urine stream.

4. _____ Pull the edge of the strip over the rim of the container you are collecting the urine in to get rid of excess urine.

5. _____ Wait 15 seconds (follow the bottle's directions for the time) and compare the ketone portion of the test strip with the ketone color chart on the test strip bottle. Or the strip may show a + or − symbol.

6. ____ Remove and dispose of your gloves in the disposable trash bag, throw the trash bag away, and wash your hands after handling each specimen.

PROCEDURE 18-8 – TESTING A STOOL SPECIMEN FOR OCCULT BLEEDING

1. ____ Put on gloves. **Note:** *If you contaminate your gloves in any way during the procedure, you must change to a new pair of gloves.*
2. ____ After the resident has a bowel movement, use an applicator to obtain a small sample of the fecal material.
3. ____ Put a thin smear of the fecal material on the kit's test slide in the designated area. Some test slides have two sections so that you can test smears from two different areas of the stool.
4. ____ After putting the smear on the slide, wait 3–5 minutes. (This allows the slide to better absorb the fecal matter.)
5. ____ Put two drops of the developer solution on the back of the slide directly behind the stool sample.
6. ____ Read the results in 60 seconds (or follow the directions in the kit). If any blue or blue–green color appears around the edge of the sample, the test is positive for occult bleeding. **Note:** *Testing is often done with three consecutive stools because bleeding may occur only at times rather than continuously. Checking three stools at different times can better identify occult bleeding.*
7. ____ Remove and dispose of your gloves in the disposable trash bag, throw the trash bag away, and wash your hands after handling each specimen.

PROCEDURE 19-1 – REMOVING A WOUND DRESSING

1. ____ Put on disposable gloves. You do not need sterile gloves to remove the dressing.
2. ____ Gently loosen the tape on the dressing, and pull the tape ends toward the wound. Holding the skin at the same time helps to prevent damage to the skin.
3. ____ Remove the old dressing and place it in an appropriate disposable bag.

PROCEDURE 19-2 – CLEANING A WOUND

1. ____ Open the sterile gloves and the sterile cleaning supplies.
2. ____ Put on gloves.
3. ____ Clean along the wound edges. Be sure to clean each side of the wound separately. Repeat using another moistened gauze or swab, until the entire wound is clean.
4. ____ Dispose of used cleaning supplies in an appropriate disposable bag.
5. ____ Pat the wound site dry with a sterile dressing sponge.

PROCEDURE 19-3 – DRESSING A WOUND

1. ____ Maintain sterile technique with the use of sterile gloves.
2. ____ Apply the appropriate dressing based on the care plan.
3. ____ Secure the dressing, using only the amount of tape (or other method) required to secure the dressing.

PROCEDURE 24-1 – BLOOD GLUCOSE MONITORING BY FINGER PRICK

1. ____ Have the person wash their hands in warm water and soap or use an alcohol wipe to cleanse the fingertip. Dry thoroughly.
2. ____ Put on disposable gloves. Turn on the glucose meter. Some meters require that the glucose test strip be inserted at this time.
3. ____ Squeeze/milk the end of the person's finger toward the fingertip. Quickly and confidently prick the person's finger using a lancing device. Continue to squeeze or "milk" the fingertip until you see a large drop of blood.
4. ____ Place the blood on the strip test area. Follow the guidelines for the specific glucose meter.
5. ____ Read and record the results. With some meters, the blood must remain on the strip as the meter times and processes the result. With other meters, the blood must be wiped off the test strip; then the strip is inserted into the meter for the final result and reading.
6. ____ Cover/clean the prick site with alcohol pad, gauze, or a tissue until the bleeding stops. If needed, then apply a Band-aid.
Note: *The better you are able to squeeze or "milk" the fingertip, the less deeply do you need to "prick" the skin. Remember: the person will have many finger pricks/sticks during their stay, and each one should be as painless, yet effective, as possible.*

PROCEDURE 24-2 – DIABETIC FOOT CARE

1. ____ Inspect the feet daily. Report to the nurse any calluses, corns, blisters, abrasions, redness, and nail abnormalities.
2. ____ Wash the feet daily in warm water, using nondrying soap.

3. ____ Dry thoroughly between the toes to prevent skin breakdown.
4. ____ Be sure the person wears well-fitting shoes and socks to prevent any pressure on the feet.
5. ____ Inspect the inside of shoes for foreign objects or areas of roughness.
6. ____ Report any injury to the nurse immediately.

PROCEDURE 24-3 – ASSISTING WITH DIAPHRAGMATIC BREATHING

1. ____ If able, have the person place one hand on the abdomen and the other hand on the middle of the chest. If the person is not able, ask the person if you can place your own hand on the abdomen to see and feel movement.
2. ____ Have the person breathe in slowly and deeply through the nose, while pushing out the abdomen as far as they can. You should be able to see, and the person should be able to feel, the abdomen push out the hand.
3. ____ Then have the person breathe out through pursed (partially closed or "puckered") lips while tightening their abdominal muscles. The person inhales in through the nose for a count of two and exhales through pursed lips for a count of four. You can help by counting this out for the person: 1, 2... 1, 2, 3, 4. You should be able to see, and the person should be able to feel, the abdomen move inward.
4. ____ With this type of breathing, you should be able to see, and the person should be able to feel, no chest movement—only movement in the abdomen.

PROCEDURE 24-4 – ASSISTING WITH DEEP BREATHING AND COUGHING

1. ____ Explain that after surgery a person needs to take deep breaths and cough. This helps to remove anesthesia and prevent the accumulation of lung secretions. Coughing and deep breathing are also important for someone who has been on bed rest for a period of time.
2. ____ When ready, ask them to take at least four diaphragmatic breaths as described in Procedure 24-3.
3. ____ Put on gloves.
4. ____ Elevate the head of the bed as much as the person can tolerate.
5. ____ Tell the person how to hold a pillow or splint over the surgical site.
6. ____ While holding the pillow, ask the person to take a deep breath, hold it for three seconds, and then exhale. Repeat this at least five times if the person can tolerate it. With the last two deep breaths, encourage the person to take a deep breath and cough as hard as possible while you hold the emesis basin to catch any sputum secretions.
7. ____ Clean up any secretions using tissues and the emesis basin. Note the color and consistency of any respiratory secretions. Report your findings to the health care team
8. ____ Instruct the person to continue the deep breathing and coughing exercises once an hour.

PROCEDURE 24-5 – ASSISTING WITH AN INCENTIVE SPIROMETER

1. ____ Clean mouthpiece using disposable alcohol wipe.
2. ____ Place the patient in a comfortable sitting or semi-Fowler's position.
   Note: *If the person has had surgery, this procedure should be done approximately 30 minutes after the patient has had pain medication. You and the nurse should coordinate and communicate medication times with this procedure. Also, have the person place the pillow on top of the incision to "splint" it if necessary.*
3. ____ Set the incentive spirometer as communicated to you by the nurse or noted in the orders or care plan. Instruct the person to exhale fully.
4. ____ Then the person should
   a. ____ Place mouthpiece into the mouth—hold lips tightly around the mouthpiece.
   b. ____ Take in a slow, easy, deep breath through the mouthpiece, trying to reach the goal by watching the ball move up in the spirometer tube
   c. ____ When the goal is reached, or if the ball will move upward no further, hold breath for three seconds
   d. ____ Remove the mouthpiece, relax and exhale.
5. ____ Encourage the person to cough.
6. ____ Praise the person's results.
7. ____ Notify the nurse if the person was not able to reach their spirometer goals.

PROCEDURE 24-6 – ADMINISTERING OXYGEN BY NASAL CANNULA

1. ____ Post no-smoking signs.
2. ____ If ordered, fill the humidifier to the appropriate level.
3. ____ Attach the connecting tube from the nasal cannula to the humidifier.
4. ____ The nurse will set the flow rate at the prescribed liters per minute.
5. ____ Assist the nurse to place the tips of the cannula in the person's nose and adjust the straps around ears for a snug, comfortable fit.

PROCEDURE 24-7 – ADMINISTERING OXYGEN BY SIMPLE FACE MASK

1. ____ Post no-smoking signs.
2. ____ Make sure the humidifier is filled to the appropriate level.
3. ____ The nurse will adjust the flow meter.
4. ____ Assist the nurse to apply the mask on the person's face and adjust the straps so the mask fits securely.
5. ____ If the tubing fills with water, drain the tubing by emptying the water. Do not drain it back into the humidifier.
6. ____ If a heating element is used, check the temperature. The humidifier bottle should be warm, not hot, to the touch.

PROCEDURE 25-1 – SHAVING THE SURGICAL SITE

1. ____ Raise the bed to a good working height.
2. ____ Assist the person to a comfortable position.
3. ____ Cover the person with the bath blanket. Fold the bed linens to the bottom of the bed.
4. ____ Place the plastic-covered pad under the person. Remove any clothing to expose only the surgical prep area.
5. ____ Put on gloves.
6. ____ Wash and lather the surgical prep site with warm water and soap, or use the surgical prep cleansing solution to clean the skin.
7. ____ Hold the skin taut with one hand. With the other hand hold the razor at a 45 degree angle to shave the hair in the area of the surgical site. Shave in the direction of hair growth using short strokes. Be careful not to cut the skin or remove moles on the skin. If using an electric razor, gently move it over the area. If using a depilatory cream, check with the nurse and read the directions on the package before applying it to the skin. Always ask for help if you are unsure how to shave a surgical site.
8. ____ Be sure to clean any excess lather and dry the person's skin when finished.

PROCEDURE 25-2 – ASSISTING WITH DEEP BREATHING AND COUGHING

1. ____ Explain that after surgery a person needs to take deep breaths and cough. This helps to remove anesthesia and prevent the accumulation of lung secretions. Coughing and deep breathing are also important for someone who has been on bed rest for a period of time.
2. ____ When ready, ask them to take at least four diaphragmatic breaths as described in Procedure 24-3.
3. ____ Put on gloves.
4. ____ Elevate the head of the bed as much as the person can tolerate.
5. ____ Tell the person how to hold a pillow or splint over the surgical site.
6. ____ While holding the pillow, ask the person to take a deep breath, hold it for three seconds, and then exhale. Repeat this at least five times if the person can tolerate it. With the last two deep breaths, encourage the person to take a deep breath and cough as hard as possible while you hold the emesis basin to catch any sputum secretions.
7. ____ Clean up any secretions using tissues and the emesis basin. Note the color and consistency of any respiratory secretions. Report your findings to the heath care team.
8. ____ Instruct the person to continue the deep breathing and coughing exercises once an hour.

PROCEDURE 26-1 – ASSISTING WITH A SITZ BATH

1. ____ Fill the Sitz bath two thirds full with warm water. Check the water temperature with a thermometer. Place the disposable Sitz bath on the toilet. You may only need to set the Sitz bath up, or to demonstrate how to fill the bath with water and place it on the toilet so that the mother can do it on her own at home.
2. ____ Put on gloves if you will be assisting with the Sitz bath.
3. ____ Assist the mother if needed, to the bathroom. Help her remove clothing and the peri-pad, and then help her onto the toilet.
4. ____ Cover her with a bath blanket.

5.   If she complains of dizziness or feeling light-headed, stay with her until she feels better and then assist her back to bed.
6.   Allow for privacy. Give her the call light.
7.   Check on her every five minutes. Allow 15 to 20 minutes total for the bath, or stop when the water becomes too cold or the mother has had enough.
8.   Assist her with washing, drying, and dressing. Help her safely return to her bed or chair if needed.

Note: *Most mothers will be able to take a Sitz bath alone.*

PROCEDURE 26-2 – DIAPERING A NEWBORN

1.   Put on gloves.
2.   Remove the diaper by lifting the plastic tabs attached to the sides of the disposable diaper, or remove the diaper pins from a cloth diaper.
3.   Wash, rinse, and dry the infant's genital area, using the same principles you learned for bathing a resident, or clean the genital area with the disposable wipe using the same principles for bathing the genital area.
4.   Clean the area around the umbilical cord with an antiseptic wipe or as ordered, if applicable.
5.   For newly circumcised male newborns only, clean and apply petroleum jelly to the head of the penis using a cotton-tipped applicator, if it was ordered. Then wrap it with a small piece of gauze.
6.   Apply a small amount of cream or lotion to the genital area and buttocks to prevent diaper rash, if used.
7.   With the clean diaper in one hand, gently grasp the infant's legs with your other hand. Raise them up enough to slide the diaper under the infant's buttocks. If using a cloth diaper, make a fold in the diaper in the front for a male infant and a fold in the back for a female; this adds extra protection where it is needed. Bring the diaper between the infant's legs.
8.   Hold the diaper snug around one hip and the abdomen, and fasten the tab snugly. Do the same for the other side. If using a cloth diaper, hold the cloth snugly with one hand while positioning the pin on each side carefully so the opening faces the infant's back. Do not pinch the infant's skin.
9.   If the infant still has the umbilical cord stump, fold down the top of the diaper.
10.   If using a cloth diaper, add a rubber pant over the diaper so the infant's clothes are not soiled. With a disposable diaper rubber pants are not needed.

    Note the color and consistency of the infant's stool. Transitional stools change from tarry black to greenish black, to greenish brown, to brownish yellow, to greenish yellow.

PROCEDURE 26-3 – BATHING A NEWBORN

1.   Put on gloves. Undress the newborn, and remove the diaper. If using disposable diapers, dispose of the diaper in the plastic trash bag; if using a cloth diaper, dispose of the diaper into the container. Take off your gloves, and discard them in the plastic trash bag. You may want to place a wash cloth over the infant's genital area in case the infant voids during bathing.

    Note: *Put on gloves if this is the infant's first bath. If not, use standard precautions as they apply to bathing. Put gloves on at the beginning of the bathing procedure if you are giving the infant a tub bath, because you use one hand to always hold the infant secure in the tub.*
2.   Check the temperature of the water. It should be at 100 to 101 degrees F. If you do not have a thermometer, use the inside of your wrist to test the water temperature. The water should be warm to the touch but not hot.
3.   Begin by bathing the infant's eyes. With the wash cloth, make a mitt as you learned in Chapter 16. Using no soap, wash one eye at a time. Be sure to wash from inside corner of the eye outward toward the infant's ear, never using the same corner of the wash cloth twice. Rinse and dry the eyes.
4.   Wash, rinse, and dry the infant's face, ears, and neck.
5.   Pick up and hold the infant as though you were holding a football in one hand. Support the infant's head in your hand and rest the body on your forearm.
6.   Holding the infant over the basin, wash the infant's head by pouring a small amount of warm water from the disposable cup over the infant's head. Do not let the water go into the infant's eyes. Place a small amount of shampoo (approximately the size of a dime) on the infant's head. Using gentle circular motions, wash the infant's head and hair. Rinse thoroughly by pouring more warm water from the cup over the infant's head. Pat dry.
7.   If you are using a tub (after the umbilical cord stump has fallen off), gently place the infant into the tub filled with warm water feet first, using both your hands with one hand supporting the upper part of the infant including the head and neck, and one hand supporting the lower part of the infant's body. Once you have placed the infant into the tub, always keep one hand securely under the infant's upper

back and shoulders to keep the infant safe. If you are not using a tub, the best way to bathe the rest of the infant's body is to lay the infant down on a clean surface.

8. ____ Wash using baby soap. If the skin is dry, use only water because the soap may dry the infant's skin more. Rinse and dry the front of the infant including the arms and hands. Clean around the umbilical cord stump, but do not get it wet.

9. ____ Wash, rinse, and dry the legs and feet.

10. ____ Carefully turn the infant over to a prone position. Wash, rinse, and dry the infant's back and buttocks. If bathing the infant in a tub, reverse the hold with your other hand holding the infant as you wash, rinse, and dry the infant's back and buttocks.

11. ____ If you are not bathing the infant in a tub, put on gloves and with a new clean wash cloth, wash, rinse, and dry the perineal area of a female by gently spreading the labia, using a different corner of the wash cloth for each downward stroke. Move from the front of the genital area back toward the rear anal area. For a male infant, wash using a new clean wash cloth from the tip of the penis down the shaft toward the scrotum. Then wash the scrotum, groin, and anal area last. Be sure to clean between the skin folds. If the male has been circumcised, follow the procedure for caring for a circumcision. If bathing the infant in the tub, using a new clean wash cloth wash and rinse the genital are using the same principles described above for male and female infants.

12. ____ With both hands lift the infant out of the tub, or place the infant after a sponge bath, onto a bath towel covering the infant's head.

13. ____ Put on a clean diaper.

14. ____ Dress the infant. Wrap the infant in the receiving blanket for warmth.

Note: *While bathing the infant, observe the skin and report any unusual findings. When bathing, move as quickly as possible so the infant does not loose unnecessary body heat.*

PROCEDURE 26-4 – CARE OF A CIRCUMCISION

1. ____ Put on gloves.

2. ____ Place the infant on the back.

3. ____ Remove the soiled diaper and dressing surrounding the tip of the penis, if one is present. Dispose of the soiled diaper and dressing in a plastic bag.

4. ____ With each diaper change, gently clean the tip of the penis with warm water and mild soap. Rinse and dry this area. Then wash and dry the rest of the perineal area.

5. ____ Put some petroleum jelly on a cotton-tipped applicator and place it on the tip of the penis. The health care professional may order a petroleum jelly gauze to be gently wrapped around the tip of the infant's penis for the first 24 to 48 hours after the procedure.

PROCEDURE 27-1 – RANGE-OF-MOTION EXERCISES

Note: *Do each exercise 5-10 times, depending on the resident's comfort level with each extremity.*

The Arm

Start with the shoulder and work your way down to the hand. For each exercise help the resident move the joint or move it yourself, depending on how much they can do independently.

The Shoulder

Place one hand under the resident's elbow and the other under their wrist. Allow the resident's forearm to rest on your body as you move the arm. If the resident is on their back, stand close to the side of the arm you are moving.

1. ____ Help the resident to lift their arm up toward the head of the bed with the elbow straight (flexion).

2. ____ Bring the arm back down to the bed (extension).

3. ____ Help the resident to lift their arm out to the side with the elbow straight (abduction)

4. ____ Bring the arm back toward the side (adduction).

5. ____ Help the resident lift their arm halfway out to the side. With the elbow bent rotate the arm down (internal rotation) and up (external rotation).

The Elbow

Place one hand above the resident's elbow and use your other hand to support the wrist. The wrist position should be neutral, not bent forward or backward.

1. ____ Help the resident bend the elbow by bringing the hand toward the upper arm with the palm facing up (flexion).
2. ____ Help the resident straighten the elbow by bringing the hand down toward the bed until the elbow is as straight as possible (extension).
3. ____ Help the resident turn their palm over with the elbow fairly straight and the wrist neutral (pronation).
4. ____ Help the resident turn their palm back up with the elbow fairly straight and the wrist neutral (supination).

The Wrist

Place one hand around the resident's forearm just above the wrist and your other hand in their hand.

1. ____ Help the resident bend their wrist down (flexion).
2. ____ Help the resident bend their wrist back (extension).
3. ____ Help the resident move their hand toward the little finger side of the wrist (ulnar deviation).
4. ____ Help the resident move their hand toward the thumb side of the wrist (radial deviation).

The Hand

Use your fingers to help the person move their fingers one by one.

1. ____ Bend and straighten each finger at each of the creases (joints of the fingers). Then curl the hand into a fist, and straighten the fingers back out (flexion and extension).
2. ____ Spread the fingers away from each other one at a time (abduction) and then back together one at a time (adduction).
3. ____ Bring each finger across the palm to the thumb and back out (opposition).

The Leg

Start with the hip and work your way down to the foot.

The Hip

Place one hand under the thigh and the other hand below the knee around the calf. Adjust your hand placement as needed to be comfortable for both you and the resident.

1. ____ Help the resident bring their leg up toward the chest with the knee bent (flexion).
2. ____ Bring their leg back down toward the bed (extension).
3. ____ Help the resident bring their leg out to the side (abduction).
4. ____ Bring their leg back toward the other leg (adduction).
5. ____ Help the resident bring the leg partly up toward the chest with the knee bent. Now gently turn the leg in (internal rotation) and out (external rotation).

The Knee

Place one hand above the resident's knee under or on their thigh and one hand below their knee around the calf.

1. ____ Help the resident bend the leg up toward the chest slightly. From this position, help them bend the knee (flexion).
2. ____ With the hip in the same position as described above, help the resident straighten the knee (extension).

The Ankle

Place one hand above the resident's ankle around the lower part of the calf and the other hand around the bottom of their foot.

1. ____ Help the resident bend the foot up toward the head while the knee is held straight (dorsiflexion), and then point the foot downward (plantarflexion).
2. ____ Help the resident turn the bottom of the foot outward (eversion) and then inward (inversion).

The Foot

As with the hand, place your fingers around each of the resident's toes and gently bend (flexion) and straighten each toe at each of the joints (extension). You can also bend and straighten all the toes at once.

PROCEDURE 27-2 - ASSISTING WITH WALKING

1. ____ Ensure that the resident is wearing shoes that fit properly before assisting with walking. Put the guard belt on the resident.
2. ____ If the resident walks without an assistive device, stand at their side so that you can watch their face as you hold onto the belt from behind. If the resident uses a walker or cane, stand on that side with one hand on the back of the belt and the other on the walker (or cane if the resident needs help with the cane). Most residents who use a cane can hold it by themselves, so you can stand on the other side. Make sure that the resident holds the cane in the correct hand.
3. ____ Walk with the resident. Have them take small steps and slowly progress to larger ones. When walking in hallways, encourage residents not using a walker to use the safety bars for added support. Always stand on their other side so they may use the bars.

(9:30) quinta